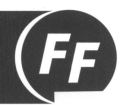

FAST FACTS

Difficulties

Indispensable
Guides to
Clinical
Practice

y and

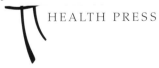

HEALTH PRESS

Oxford

Fast Facts – Specific Learning Difficulties
First published November 2003

Text © 2003 Amanda Kirby, Bonnie J Kaplan
© 2003 in this edition Health Press Limited
Health Press Limited, Elizabeth House, Queen Street, Abingdon,
Oxford OX14 3JR, UK
Tel: +44 (0)1235 523233
Fax: +44 (0)1235 523238

Book orders can be placed by telephone or via the website.
For regional distributors or to order via the website, please go to:
www.fastfacts.com
For telephone orders, please call 01752 202301 (UK) or
1 800 538 1287 (North America, toll free).

Fast Facts is a trademark of Health Press Limited.

A CIP catalogue record for this title is available from the British Library.

ISBN 1-903734-39-8

Kirby A (Amanda)
Fast Facts – Specific Learning Difficulties/
Amanda Kirby, Bonnie J Kaplan

Typesetting and page layout by Zed, Oxford, UK.

Printed by Fine Print (Services) Ltd, Oxford, UK.

Printed with vegetable inks on fully biodegradable and
recyclable paper manufactured from sustainable forests.

444   001
Low emissions
during production

Low
chlorine

Sustainable
forests

Glossary 4

Introduction 5

General issues of diagnosis and treatment 7

Dyslexia (reading disability) 15

Developmental coordination disorder (dyspraxia) 24

Attention deficit hyperactivity disorder 31

Oppositional defiant disorder and conduct disorder 41

Asperger's syndrome 50

Obsessive–compulsive disorder 60

Future trends 67

Useful addresses 69

Index 73

Glossary of abbreviations and synonyms

ADD: attention deficit disorder, also called ADHD

ADHD: attention deficit hyperactivity disorder

ASDI: Asperger Syndrome (and high-functioning autism) Diagnostic Interview

CAST: Childhood Asperger Syndrome Test

CD: conduct disorder

DCD: developmental coordination disorder, called dyspraxia in the UK

DEST: Dyslexia Early Years Screening Test

DISCO: Diagnostic Interview for Social and Communication Disorders

DSM-IV: *Diagnostic and Statistical Manual of Mental Disorders* of the American Psychiatric Association, fourth edition

DST: Dyslexia Screening Test

dyslexia: usually called reading disability in North America

dyspraxia: called developmental coordination disorder in North America

OCD: obsessive–compulsive disorder

ODD: oppositional defiant disorder

PECS: Picture Exchange Communication System

reading disability: called dyslexia in the UK

SENCO: special educational needs coordinator

TEACH: Teaching and Education of Autistic Children and Handicapped Children

WIAT-II: Wechsler Individual Achievement Test II

WISC III: Wechsler Intelligence Scale for Children, version III

WJ–R: Woodcock–Johnson Psychoeducational Battery – revised

Introduction

The term 'specific learning difficulties' is not universally accepted, but is commonly used to refer to three problems:
- dyslexia (usually called reading disability in North America)
- developmental coordination disorder (DCD), called dyspraxia in the UK
- attention deficit hyperactivity disorder (ADHD), also called attention deficit disorder (ADD).

In addition, four other conditions commonly overlap with these learning and attention problems:
- oppositional defiant disorder (ODD)
- conduct disorder (CD)
- Asperger's syndrome
- obsessive–compulsive disorder (OCD).

Fast Facts – Specific Learning Difficulties considers these six learning and behavior problems, addressing four questions for each.
- What is this disorder, including its core symptoms and signs, what is its incidence and prevalence, and what is known about its cause?
- What are the criteria for this disorder as specified by the *Diagnostic and Statistical Manual of Mental Disorders*, 4th edition, of the American Psychiatric Association (*DSM-IV*)?
- Who assesses and diagnoses this disorder, and how?
- What are the treatments for this disorder, including management at home and in school?

Key reference

American Psychiatric Association. *Diagnostic and Statistical Manual of Mental Disorders (DSM-IV)*, 4th edn. Washington, DC: American Psychiatric Association, 1994.

Advantages and disadvantages of labeling children

The use of a diagnostic label to characterize a child makes many people uncomfortable, and indeed, in many situations children themselves may be better off if they are not told about their diagnosis and labeling. In the current era, however, labeling is a necessity and can even be beneficial (Table 1.1).

Of course, labels may also be harmful in certain ways. For example, a label can have negative connotations that may affect individuals who come into contact with the labeled child. Some people may have preconceived ideas about a disorder based on their previous experience of others with the same label, such as a child with Asperger's syndrome

---

TABLE 1.1

Advantages of diagnostic labels for specific learning difficulties

- Acknowledges for parents that there is a genuine reason for their worries and concerns

- Renders parents less likely to be dismissed by others as just 'over-anxious parents'

- Can make funds or services available to the child; in some settings, the absence of a label means that funding will not be allocated for that child

- Can legitimize a genuine condition: e.g. for many years, dyslexia was erroneously seen as a 'middle-class' condition, a label used by parents to excuse the poor academic performance of their children

- Allows children to be counted for research purposes

- Can assist others who work with the child to focus on the appropriate type of intervention

- May be used as a legal reference point to consider one child's support compared with others

- May be used by authorities to plan service delivery

- Helps in determining the appropriate baseline assessment to be used before school remediation programs

who may have been seen as a difficult child rather than a child with difficulties. In addition, a child may be given more than one label or even the wrong label, or may view the label as a stigma for life that implies disability rather than as a difficulty/difficulties that can improve.

Overlapping conditions

Many, if not most, children with a developmental problem qualify for more than one diagnostic label. For example, a population study showed that 23% of children showed signs of developmental coordination disorder (DCD), 8% met criteria for attention deficit hyperactivity disorder (ADHD), and 19% were categorized as dyslexic. Nearly 25% of the affected children were found to have all three, while 10% had both ADHD and DCD, and 22% had dyslexia and DCD. In another population study, 87% of children meeting the full criteria for ADHD had one or more diagnoses and 67% at least two additional diagnoses. The most common additional diagnoses were oppositional defiant disorder (ODD) and DCD.

Much of the literature on this issue uses the term 'comorbidity', intended to convey the idea that two or more conditions occur together. The term comorbidity is not appropriate in this situation, however, at least partly because the assumption that the multiple disorders have independent etiologies cannot be proved. In fact, the very high overlap of developmental disorders may be an indication that they are not independent. A new conceptual framework, which has been called atypical brain development, may help to explain developmental disorders and their relationship to each other. One implication of this framework is a new emphasis on the individual strengths and weaknesses of each child, with individualized treatment programs based on the child's profile rather than on a diagnostic category.

The present book makes no assumptions about the independence of the six categories of disorders discussed and emphasizes the importance of individual assessments and treatment recommendations.

Diagnostic labels versus functional labels

In view of the disadvantages of labeling mentioned above, and because children do not fit into the neat diagnostic boxes specified in the

DSM-IV, the concept of atypical brain development has some tempting features. For example, it implies that children would be better served if we abandoned *diagnostic* labels and instead provided *functional* descriptions of strengths and weaknesses (Table 1.2).

Approach to assessment/diagnosis

A proper and detailed assessment of a child's profile of neurodevelopmental strengths and difficulties is a critical step in devising an effective management plan at home and in school. The following general principles can guide the assessment process.

- Health professionals and educators need to understand the key specific learning difficulties and have some understanding of the underlying mechanisms of function.
- The assessment process should stress the search for each child's strengths as well as outline the difficulties so that practical help or remediation can be provided as appropriate.
- Information should be gathered through a process of formal testing and clinical observations and gathered from a number of viewpoints, for example from home, school, and the children's clinic or children's center (a multidisciplinary focused assessment and treatment center), to ensure an objective diagnosis and a complete differential diagnosis, and that no underlying neurological disorder, for example epilepsy, muscular dystrophy or cerebral palsy, has been missed.

TABLE 1.2

Examples of diagnostic and functional labels for specific learning difficulties

Diagnostic label	Functional label
• DCD	• Difficulty with ball skills and handwriting
• ADHD	• Difficulty staying on task, impulsive behavior
• Dyslexia	• Spelling, reading difficulties
• Asperger's syndrome	• Difficulty with social relationships

Depending on the complexity of the child's difficulties, the assessments should be made in several stages, by an interdisciplinary team if possible. First, observations from parents and teachers should be sought, providing them with some guidance in the areas of information required. This should be followed by evaluation by a health professional to consider any underlying neurological causes for dysfunction, and by an interdisciplinary team working together in time and place so that a cohesive and complete assessment is made and all underlying features have been considered before diagnosis. The final evaluation should be at school or in the community, to gain further information or confirm the diagnosis, as well as to communicate and plan the remediation programs.

It is important to seek patterns that are evident in the observation and/or tests of more than one individual and across time. The behavior or development of children with suspected specific learning difficulties should differ significantly from those of their peers to justify a diagnosis. Developmental milestones as markers of age-appropriate actions in language and motor development can be useful.

Approach to management

The successful management of a child with specific learning difficulties requires a multifaceted, coordinated approach. The parents, teachers, and all healthcare professionals involved need to seek common goals for the child and must communicate these among themselves. This is one of the most difficult aspects of management, as assessment may be completed at different times and in different places, making good communication hard to achieve. At present, there are also differing levels of understanding and expectation of what health professionals can offer in terms of therapeutic intervention, what the education system is able to give in terms of manpower and resources, and who is responsible for payment and delivery.

The result of a multidisciplinary assessment should be a jargon-free report on the child, with an individually tailored program of support for the child's unique needs.

- A good report should highlight points at which a strategy could be employed to bypass a difficulty that cannot be entirely overcome, for example the use of a laptop computer for writing problems.
- It should also show the steps required to achieve improvement and how improvement should be measured.
- It should indicate where difficulties may arise in the future and when a review of the child's progress may be required.
- It should indicate whether further assessment by other agencies is required.

Associated problems, such as peer relationships, low self-esteem and family dysfunction, should be specifically addressed in the individualized management plan.

Available help

Local specialist services. After the primary care team has gathered as much information as possible from parents and school (if the child is of school age) and undertaken a basic developmental assessment, it can then refer a child to local children's services (Table 1.3). Waiting lists in different areas may vary considerably, from a few weeks to a

---

TABLE 1.3

Local specialist services

A child with a suspected specific learning difficulty may be referred from the primary care team to any of these other local services

- Pediatrician or pediatric neurologist, often needed for a differential diagnosis

- Speech and language therapist, to evaluate expressive or receptive language difficulties as well as pragmatic language dysfunction, social and communication difficulties

- Physiotherapist, to assess gross motor difficulties, postural difficulties

- Occupational therapist, to assess fine motor skills or difficulties related to developmental coordination disorder

- Clinical psychologist, to evaluate and advise on behavior management and social difficulties

few years for some services. Basic practical advice to parents in the interim can be extremely useful to reduce anxiety and help the child become more able.

Local educational services.

In the UK, parents can contact their local education authorities or local government body (for example the National Assembly of Wales) for further advice on their statutory rights, and for additional help and provision for their children. Information on codes of practice is also posted on government websites. These codes of practice differ in different areas, but always delineate the type of help that should be provided as a statutory right and the complaint/appeal process if parents are unhappy with what a child is currently receiving.

In most schools, the first person to approach is the classroom teacher, followed by the special needs coordinator (known in the UK as the SENCO), who can usually give advice on the type of help the child may need, and whether the child requires further assessment. The school can arrange for assessments by the educational psychologist or can refer the child for additional assessments to ascertain the educational need and support required to remedy the difficulties.

Several voluntary organizations, for example SNAP Cymru in Wales and Network 81 in England (see 'Useful addresses' at the back of this book), can deliver additional, independent help to parents. These organizations will advise parents on how to proceed and can provide information sheets on many educational areas.

In North America, parents can first contact the classroom teacher to determine what resources are available for evaluation and assistance. In some situations, this approach will be sufficient to enable parents to obtain an assessment of their child's abilities. The resources of the school system will determine whether such an evaluation will result in individual financial costs for the family.

If a classroom teacher is not sufficiently helpful, it may be useful for the family to approach the school principal and/or special needs coordinator. Some school systems have an office specifically to help families of children with special needs.

An excellent resource for any family just encountering the concept and challenge of learning problems in their children is their local chapter of the Learning Disabilities Association. Contact information for both the USA and Canada can be found at the end of this book.

Parent support organizations. Each condition described in this book has its own voluntary support organization(s), whose addresses are given in a section at the end of this book. Many of the organizations have a range of leaflets and books available, some have telephone support lines, and some provide assessment and treatment services for individuals. As children often have overlapping conditions, however, so parent support groups often have many similarities. In some geographical areas, some groups will be stronger than others.

Key points – General issues of diagnosis and treatment

- Diagnostic labels can validate the presence of a specific learning disorder and help in planning appropriate intervention, but may also stigmatize a child for life.
- Because many children with a developmental problem qualify for more than one diagnostic label, it may be more appropriate to use a functional label which focuses on individual strengths and weaknesses.
- Assessment and diagnosis of a child with a specific learning difficulty requires a multidisciplinary approach, in which parents, school and community organizations participate in addition to primary and secondary care specialists.
- Successful management requires a coordinated approach, with good communication between parents, teachers and healthcare professionals to achieve common goals identified in an individualized management plan.
- Parents of children with specific learning difficulties can obtain help and support from local specialist services, local educational services and parent support organizations.

Key references

Armitage M, Larkin D. Laterality, motor asymmetry and clumsiness in children. *Hum Movement Sci* 1993; 12:155–77.

Burton A, Miller D. Assessing movement skill and concept learning. In: *Physical Education Methods for Classroom Teachers*. Champaign, IL: Human Kinetics Publications, 1999:109.

Cratty BJ. *Clumsy Child Syndromes: Descriptions, Evaluation, and Remediation*. Langhorne, PA: Harwood, 1994.

Gilger JW, Kaplan BJ. Atypical brain development: a conceptual framework for understanding developmental learning disabilities. *Dev Neuropsychol* 2001;20:465–81.

Harvey WJ, Reid G. Motor performance of children with attention-deficit hyperactivity disorder: A preliminary investigation. *Adapt Phys Act Q* 1997;14:189–202.

Henderson SE, Barnett AL. The classification of specific motor coordination disorders in children: some problems to be solved. *Hum Movement Sci* 1998;17:449–70.

Kadesjo B, Gillberg C. The comorbidity of ADHD in the general population of Swedish school-age children. *J Child Psychol Psychiatry* 2001;42:487–92.

Kaplan BJ, Dewey D, Crawford S, Wilson B. The term 'comorbidity' is of questionable value in reference to developmental disorders: Data and theory. *J Learn Disabil* 2001;34: 555–565.

Landgren M, Pettersson R, Kjellman B, Gillberg C. ADHD, DAMP and other neurodevelopmental/psychiatric disorders in 6-year-old children: epidemiology and co-morbidity. *Dev Med Child Neurol* 1996;38:891–906.

Landgren M, Kjellman B, Gillberg C. Attention deficit disorder with developmental coordination disorders. *Arch Dis Child* 1998;79:207–12.

Levine MD. *Educational Care: a System for Understanding and Helping Children with Learning Problems at Home and in School*. Cambridge, MA: Educators Publishing Service, 1994.

Martini R, Heath N, Missiuna C. A North American analysis of the relationship between learning disability and developmental coordination disorder. *Int J Spec Educ* 1999;14:46–58.

Pryde KM, Roy EA. Mechanisms of developmental coordination disorders: individual analyses and disparate findings. *Brain Cogn* 1999;40:230–4.

In the UK, dyslexia is considered to be difficulty in the acquisition of reading, writing and spelling skills; in North America it has recently been defined more narrowly as 'a specific language-based disorder of constitutional origin characterized by difficulties in single-word decoding, usually reflecting insufficient phonological processing abilities.' There is general agreement that dyslexia reflects a constitutional or congenital problem, and is not the result of social or emotional difficulties, physical handicaps, inadequate teaching, or limited intelligence. It may be caused by a combination of phonological, auditory and visual processing difficulties. Working memory, semantic access and speed of processing may also be affected. Despite first being described in 1878 by a German physician, Dr Kussmaul, who referred to a man unable to learn to read as having 'word blindness', dyslexia is still the subject of much debate on its identification and the best method of intervention.

Estimates of its prevalence vary according to the definition of dyslexia and the way in which it is assessed. The British Dyslexia Association suggests that 4% of the population will be severely dyslexic, requiring support at school and beyond, and a further 6% may have mild or moderate dyslexia. Different studies offer different percentages owing to the diverse cut-off criteria used. Some reports suggest that up to four times as many boys as girls are dyslexic. However, it is now acknowledged that this may be a function of the method of referral; that is, when failing, a boy is more likely than a girl to be disruptive in class, and therefore to be recognized as needing outside help. Furthermore, girls' language skills exceed boys' throughout most of school, and since a single (genderless) set of tests is used, boys are naturally more likely to appear as failing.

Etiology

It was reported over 50 years ago that if one parent has dyslexia, each child has about a 46% probability of displaying the same problem.

Since then, the genetic predisposition for reading difficulties has become increasingly clear, and current heritability estimates for various reading phenotypes are quite high, ranging from 0.51 to 0.93.

Although the first molecular genetic studies appeared in 1983, specific predisposing genes for dyslexia have not yet been isolated. Several chromosomal regions have been intensively studied, however, particularly two areas of chromosome 6 and regions of chromosomes 1, 2 and 15. Current genetic linkage research tends to support the idea that a number of genes at different loci, rather than a single locus, may contribute to the range of reading abilities/disabilities.

Pathophysiology

There is now a general consensus that the central deficit experienced by poor readers is related to phonologic processing. Much research also suggests that there is a general impairment in the ability to perform skills automatically, which is thought by some to be dependent in part on the cerebellum, although recent investigations suggest otherwise. In addition, there is evidence that some individuals with dyslexia have a 'fault' with the magnocellular neurons in the brain (responsible for processing rapidly changing information in the auditory and visual systems) that influences sensory processing.

Long-term outcome

Dyslexia has been estimated to affect 10–50% of the adult prison populations. There may, however, be social and cultural reasons for reading disabilities, reflected in the higher estimates. A recent Swedish study reported 11% of the prison population having severe difficulties, which is more consistent with the general population.

Recent research suggests that individuals with dyslexia exhibit significantly higher rates of all internalizing and externalizing disorders than those without dyslexia. People with better language skills may have a better outcome than those with additional language difficulties.

Signs and symptoms

Dyslexia usually presents around the age of 7–8 years as the child's deficiencies become clear in the school setting (Table 2.1, Figure 2.1).

TABLE 2.1

Common signs of dyslexia

- Hesitant and inaccurate reading
- Need to re-read materials to gain an understanding
- Difficulty with sequences, e.g. putting dates in order
- Erratic spelling
- Reversal of letters (occurs in many normally developing children at times)
- Auditory language problems or visual–spatial problems (may contribute to difficulties with reading and spelling)
- Inability to distinguish sounds or shapes on the page

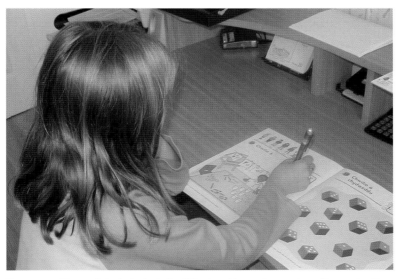

Figure 2.1 Signs of dyslexia include difficulty with reading and spelling and with sequences, and inability to distinguish sounds or shapes on the page.

Often there are other associated symptoms, such as poor spelling and handwriting, and occasionally mathematical difficulties. The *DSM-IV* criteria for a diagnosis of dyslexia are given in Table 2.2.

Assessment. Traditionally, dyslexia has been seen as an educational problem. Most health professionals had little knowledge of it and did

TABLE 2.2

DSM-IV criteria for a diagnosis of dyslexia

- Reading achievement, as measured by individually administered standardized tests of reading accuracy or comprehension, is substantially below that expected given the person's chronological age, measured intelligence and age-appropriate education
- The disturbance in the first criterion significantly interferes with academic achievement or activities of daily living that require reading skills
- If a sensory deficit is present, the reading difficulties are in excess of those usually associated with the specific sensory deficit

not place it in their therapeutic province. If dyslexia is seen as a developmental language disorder, however (Figure 2.2), the role of the health professional becomes increasingly important, and this shift may affect speech and language remediation services in the future.

Assessment is usually carried out by an educational psychologist after a referral from the parent or teacher. The referral often happens when the child's reading skills have begun to fall behind those of peers. The educational psychologist performs a battery of tests to identify where the difficulty lies and to recommend an appropriate school-based remediation program. Standardized measures, such as the Wechsler Intelligence Scale for Children, version III (WISC III), are used to assess

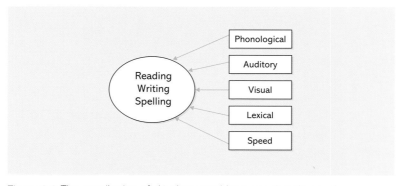

Figure 2.2 The contribution of developmental language disorders to the educational difficulties of children with dyslexia.

general intellectual ability. In addition, educational psychologists in the UK use other more specific tools, such as the Dyslexia Early Years Screening Test (DEST) for early years testing, the Dyslexia Screening Test (DST), and the Aston Index. The outcome from such assessment often assists teachers in defining remediation programs. In Canada and the United States, children are more typically assessed with other reading measures, such as the Wechsler Individual Achievement Test II (WIAT-II) or the Woodcock–Johnson Psychoeducational Battery – Revised (WJ–R).

The educational psychologist investigates whether the child has a semantic difficulty (does not understand the meaning of words) or a problem with phoneme segmentation (cannot see or hear the components and then put them together to create meaning and to spell the words; Table 2.3). The child's learning deficits may be attributable to:

- the visual system (not being able to recognize shape and form): this may have a visual perceptual component, and some children have figure–ground difficulties (difficulty discriminating between the print and the background)
- reading speed
- reading accuracy
- reading comprehension
- phoneme segmentation.

It is also important to identify language difficulties, whether receptive, expressive or pragmatic, which may be the underlying cause of the reading and spelling difficulties, as well as any hearing difficulties the child may have, especially at the stage of language acquisition. This

TABLE 2.3

Examples of different types of phoneme segmentation error

- **Phonetic error:**   *lap* instead of *lip*
- **Visual error:**   *lite* instead of *light*
- **Auditory error:**   *pig* instead of *big*
- **Sequential error:**   *filght* instead of *flight*

may require audiometry as well as an assessment by a speech and language therapist to consider these difficulties and to put in place remediation programs integrated into education.

Treatment

Treatment for dyslexia is usually multisensory, using visual, auditory and kinesthetic routes to reinforce learning. Once the area of difficulty is understood, the intervention is tailored to it. Favorable outcomes are dependent on the initial severity of the condition, as well as on the presence of supportive home and school environments. Treatment is often phonic-based, addressing the problem of phoneme segmentation.

TABLE 2.4

Suggestions for parents of children with dyslexia

- Have your child assessed by an educational psychologist. This will provide you with a report detailing the child's weaknesses and the help needed

- Speak to the class teacher with whom you have regular contact and who can give you regular feedback. Don't wait until parents' evening to discover that your child is not coping. Ask what you can do to help your child at home. Many schools have a special needs coordinator who will be able to offer advice

- Help your child to be more organized. Keep a copy of the class timetable at hand so that you know what subjects are being taught and when

- Support your child with homework; ensure that the task in hand is understood. See that the work is set at a level at which your child can succeed. This may mean going back a couple of stages to make sure the foundation skills are in place

- If progress is slow, encourage your child to use a computer to organize work. Make sure it has a spell-checker program; programs that help your child to spell are also available. Voice-activated software is not always helpful for younger children

- Praise your child for any amount of work they produce and for the content, even if the spelling is poor. Remember that your child is putting in far more effort than other children the same age. Positively reinforcing effort will motivate your child to do even better

If dyslexia is identified before a child is 7–8 years old and is mild to moderate (as it is in 80% of all children with these difficulties), there is some evidence that remediation programs in the classroom situation can be successful. Parents can be encouraged to help their child with the suggestions listed in Table 2.4. When the difficulties are not identified or are more severe, however, the level of help required increases greatly.

Some studies have suggested that colored lenses or overlays can make reading easier for some, but not all, children. However, the evidence is inconclusive.

Key points – Dyslexia

- Dyslexia is a reading disorder characterized by difficulties with reading speed, accuracy and/or comprehension, despite adequate intelligence and teaching.
- Up to 12% of children may suffer dyslexia, depending on how it is defined and assessed, with boys more commonly affected than girls.
- Genetic factors are involved in the etiology of dyslexia, but no specific predisposing genes have yet been isolated.
- Assessment is usually carried out by an educational psychologist using a battery of tests to identify the difficulty and to recommend an appropriate school-based remediation program.
- Treatment for dyslexia is usually multisensory, using visual, auditory and kinesthetic routes to reinforce learning.

Key references

Beitchman JH, Young AR. Learning disorders with a special emphasis on reading disorders: a review of the past 10 years. *J Am Acad Child Adolesc Psychiatry* 1997;36:1020–32.

Blachman BA. *Foundations of Reading Acquisition and Dyslexia: Implications for Early Intervention.* Mahwah, NJ: L Erlbaum Associates, 1997.

Fisher SE, Stein JF, Monaco AP. A genome-wide search strategy for identifying quantitative trait loci involved in reading and spelling disability (developmental dyslexia). *Am J Hum Genet* 1999;64:146–56.

Grigorenko EL. Developmental dyslexia: an update on genes, brains, and environments. *J Child Psychol Psychiatry* 2001;42:91–125.

Hallgren B. Specific dyslexia ('congenital word-blindness'): a clinical and genetic study. *Acta Psychiatr Scand* 1950;65(suppl): 1–287.

Katusic SK, Colligan RC, Barbaresi WJ et al. Incidence of reading disability in a population-based birth cohort, 1976–1982, Rochester, Minn. *Mayo Clin Proc* 2001;76:1081–92.

Kirk J, Reid G. An examination of the relationship between dyslexia and offending in young people and the implications for the training system. *Dyslexia* 2001;7:77–84.

Nicolson, RI, Fawcett AJ, Dean P. Developmental dyslexia: the cerebellar deficit hypothesis. *Trends Neurosci* 2001;24:508–11.

Oakland T, Black JL, Stanford G et al. An evaluation of the dyslexia training program: a multisensory method for promoting reading in students with reading disabilities. *J Learn Disabil* 1998;31:140–7.

Petryshen TL, Kaplan BJ, Liu MF et al. Evidence for a susceptibility locus (DYX4) on chromosome 6q influencing phonological coding dyslexia. *Am J Med Genet Neuropsychiatric Genet* 2001;105: 507–17.

Rae C, Harasty JA, Dzendrowskyj TE et al. Cerebellar morphology in developmental dyslexia. *Neuropsychologia* 2002;40:1285–92.

Ramus F, Pidgeon E, Frith U. The relationship between motor control and phonology in dyslexic children. *J Child Psychol Psychiatry* 2003;44:712–22.

Smythe I, Everatt J. Dyslexia diagnosis in different languages. In: Peer L, Reid G, eds. *Multilingualism, Literacy and Dyslexia.* London: David Fulton Publishers, 2000.

Snowling MJ. From language to reading and dyslexia. *Dyslexia* 2001; 7:37–46.

Stanovich KE, Siegel LS. The phenotypic performance profile of reading-disabled children: A regression-based test of the phonological-core variable-difference model. *J Educ Psychol* 1994;86:24–53.

Stein J. The magnocellular theory of developmental dyslexia. *Dyslexia* 2001;7:12–36.

Svensson I, Lundberg I, Jacobson C. The prevalence of reading and spelling difficulties among inmates of institutions for compulsory care of juvenile delinquents. *Dyslexia* 2001:7:62–76.

Motor and coordination skills are not distributed evenly across the population. While most of us master the basic movements required in life, some exceptional people become elite athletes, and others never achieve competence in fundamental gross and fine motor skills, or fail to develop good balance. Those individuals who are clumsy, whose handwriting is significantly impaired, or who exhibit other major weaknesses in motor and coordination skills are now generally diagnosed as having developmental coordination disorder (DCD).

Children with coordination and motor problems have received many different labels across the decades, across geographic boundaries, and across disciplines. Historically, such problems were described as 'clumsiness syndrome', but recently the American Psychiatric Association assigned them to the category of a disorder with the name DCD. In the UK, the term dyspraxia has often been used as an umbrella term for children with coordination difficulties. In North America, however, the term dyspraxia is seldom used at all; when it is, it usually refers to impairment of motor planning and gestures. North American research on DCD has generally focused on coordination difficulties and considered the motor planning as a part of the whole developmental disorder. To further complicate the terminology, occupational therapists in the UK have used the term dyspraxia to refer specifically to deficits in motor planning accompanied by perceptual problems, and not to mean the more general concept of coordination difficulties.

DCD is a common condition, present in about 5% of school-age children, though a recent comprehensive study suggests that moderate-to-severe DCD may be present in over 7% of 7-year-olds, with a boy:girl ratio of 5.3:1.

Etiology and pathophysiology

The changing names for DCD reflect another important problem: the underlying etiology for motor coordination difficulties is not known.

There are certainly several different subgroups. Some children given the label of DCD may have a neuromuscular or hypotonic problem, and/or a myotonic, myopathic or connective tissue disorder. They may also have a degenerative condition or a storage disorder. Ligamentous laxity presents in some children with motor-based difficulties and may be a variant or a mild form of Ehlers–Danlos syndrome (type III, congenital hypermobility syndrome). Another group seen clinically are those children who have neuromas or café-au-lait spots, who could have a variant of neurofibromatosis (NF1).

Long-term outcome

In the past, the significance of motor and coordination difficulties was not given a great deal of attention in either health or education. The long-term consequences of having these difficulties was also not considered extensively until the past few years. It is understandable that parents and teachers concerned primarily with academic success would overlook a child's failure to ride a bicycle or excel at football.

There is strong empirical evidence that the motor problems of children with DCD persist at least into adolescence and lead to the development of secondary issues of physical health, mental health and education, including poor physical fitness, poor social competence, academic problems, behavioral problems and low self-esteem.

Signs and symptoms

The most typical difficulties identified by parents and schools are shown in Table 3.1. Poor motor performance is often found alongside academic performance deficits. Some teachers and parents recognize that effective purposeful movements are a crucial part of a child's school and home life. In primary school, actions such as writing, drawing and playing are part of everyday functioning, while in secondary school, fast handwriting, keyboard skills and games are also part of everyday life. At home, self-help skills are essential to gain independence. It should be remembered, however, that the manifestations of this disorder vary with age and development. For example, younger children may display clumsiness and delays in achieving developmental motor milestones, such as walking, crawling,

TABLE 3.1

Typical difficulties experienced by children with DCD

Identified by parents	Identified by school
• Dressing	• Writing
• Eating	• Using scissors
• Doing activities under time pressure	• Puzzle activities
• Riding a bike	• Changing for physical education
	• Ball skills
	• Running

sitting, tying shoelaces (Figure 3.1), buttoning shirts or zipping pants, while older children may display difficulties with the motor aspects of assembling puzzles, building models, playing ball and printing or writing. Adults may have fewer fine motor difficulties but may be left with handwriting and organizational difficulties.

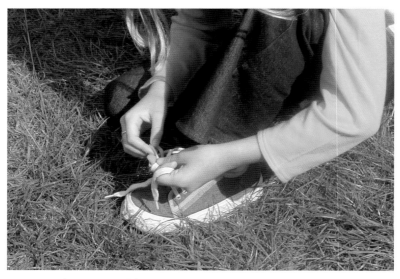

Figure 3.1 Children with DCD may have difficulty learning tasks that require fine motor control, such as tying shoelaces.

The poor performance demonstrated by children with DCD can be due to problems in planning or execution. Thus, some children with DCD have problems organizing, sequencing and generally planning movement, while others have difficulty in actual motor control. In reality it is often difficult to separate planning from execution, and many children have problems in both areas.

DCD is often found in association with other disorders, such as dyslexia. As many as 55% of those with DCD have a reading disability, and more than 40% may also have ADHD. Other secondary problems are common, with a higher incidence of behavior disorders, self-concept problems and learning difficulties than predicted from assessments of intelligence. The defining characteristic of children with DCD, however, is a motor coordination disorder, which may or may not be accompanied by any number of additional symptoms and overlapping disorders (Table 3.2, Figure 3.2).

Assessment. The child may first be identified as having difficulties by the school and is then usually referred to an educational psychologist. If there is concern, the school or education system may request further testing from occupational therapy or other services. An alternative route for assessment is through a local children's center, where a pediatrician may ask for evaluation by an occupational therapist.

TABLE 3.2

DSM-IV criteria for a diagnosis of DCD

- A marked impairment in the development of motor coordination
- The diagnosis is made only if this impairment significantly interferes with academic achievement or activities of daily living
- The diagnosis is made if the coordination difficulties are not due to a general medical condition, e.g. cerebral palsy, hemiplegia or muscular dystrophy, and the criteria are not met for pervasive developmental disorder
- If mental retardation is present, the motor difficulties are in excess of those usually associated with it

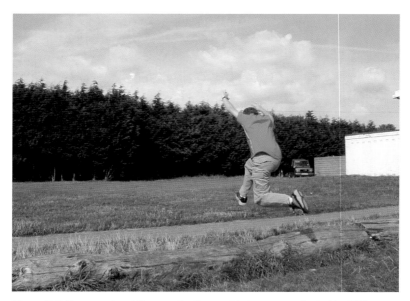

Figure 3.2 Gross motor skills, coordination and balance are affected in DCD.

The criteria used and testing performed to elicit the diagnosis vary from profession to profession. There is no true benchmarking at present. In general, local occupational therapists are likely to have their own preferred assessment tools that define the extent of the motor deficits.

It is important that any assessment information obtained is passed from health experts to educators and fits in with the curriculum, so that the teacher can help the child in school appropriately.

Treatment

A tailored approach that meets the needs of the individual child and is carried out by teachers and parents can be effective in helping children with DCD. Parents can help as suggested in Table 3.3; further assistance may be given through occupational therapy and physiotherapy. Cognitive behavioral therapy has been used effectively in some children. Motor programs are being introduced into schools to provide integrated help for the child in school.

TABLE 3.3

Suggestions for parents of children with DCD

- Provide suitable tools to help with difficult tasks, such as adapted scissors (long-looped), a computer to use instead of handwriting, organizational techniques

- Work on gross motor strength: introduce suitable sports such as swimming, riding, canoeing, walking, badminton

- Maintain self-esteem: look at hobbies that your child will enjoy, such as cookery, photography, gardening

- Maintain good liaison with the school, so that there is a parent–school partnership

---

Key points – Developmental coordination disorder

- Individuals who are clumsy, whose handwriting is significantly impaired, or who exhibit other major weaknesses in motor and coordination skills are now generally diagnosed as having DCD (also called dyspraxia, and previously known as clumsiness syndrome).
- DCD is a common condition, present in about 5% of school-age children, with more boys affected than girls.
- The underlying etiology for motor coordination difficulties is not known, though some children may have a neuromuscular or hypotonic problem, and/or a myotonic, myopathic or connective tissue disorder.
- Assessment is usually performed by an educational psychologist after referral by the school; further testing from occupational therapy or other services may also be requested.
- The criteria used and testing performed to elicit the diagnosis vary from profession to profession, and there is no true benchmarking at the present time.
- Treatment may be carried out by teachers and parents, through occupational therapy and physiotherapy; cognitive behavioral therapy and motor programs can also be effective.

Key references

Barnett AL, Kooistra L, Henderson SE. "Clumsiness" as syndrome and symptom. *Hum Movement Sci* 1998;17:435–47.

Dewey D. What is developmental dyspraxia? *Brain Cogn* 1995;29:254–74.

Gillberg IC, Gillberg C. Children with preschool minor neurodevelopmental disorders IV: Behaviour and school achievement at age 13. *Dev Med Child Neurol* 1989;31:3–13.

Gillberg IC, Gillberg C, Groth J. Children with preschool minor neurodevelopmental disorders V: Neurodevelopmental profiles at age 13. *Dev Med Child Neurol* 1989;31:14–24.

Hellgren L, Gillberg C, Gillberg IC, Enerskog I. Children with deficits in attention, motor control and perception (DAMP) almost grown up: general health at 16 years. *Dev Med Child Neurol* 1993;35:881–92.

Kadesjo B, Gillberg C. Attention deficits and clumsiness in Swedish 7-year-old children. *Dev Med Child Neurol* 1998;40:796–804.

Kaplan BJ, Wilson BN, Dewey D, Crawford SG. DCD may not be a discrete disorder. *Hum Movement Sci* 1998;17:471–490.

Missiuna C, Polatajko H. Developmental dyspraxia by any other name: are they all just clumsy children? *Am J Occup Ther* 1995;49:619–27.

Polatajko HJ, Mandich A, Miller LT, Macnab JJ. Cognitive orientation to daily occupational performance: part II – the evidence. *Phys Occup Ther Pediatr* 2001;20:83–106.

Stephenson E, McKay C, Chesson R. An investigative study of early developmental factors in children with motor/learning difficulties. *Br J Occup Ther* 1990;53:4–6.

Sugden DA, Chambers ME. Intervention approaches and children with developmental coordination disorder. *Pediatr Rehabil* 1998;2:139–47.

Attention deficit hyperactivity disorder (ADHD or ADD) has been recognized since ancient Greek times, but the label for this behavioral syndrome has varied enormously through the ages. The current designation from the American Psychiatric Association *DSM-IV* is ADHD, though the public often continues to use the term ADD. The *DSM-IV* specifies three subtypes of ADHD:

- primarily inattentive
- hyperactive–impulsive
- combined inattentive and hyperactive–impulsive.

ADHD is part of a spectrum of specific learning difficulties. It is not correlated with intelligence, and contrary to common belief, IQ is normally distributed in children with ADHD; there is no association with giftedness. Also contrary to common belief, memory is not unusually weak in these children. If children with ADHD attend to information, they remember it just as well as other children do.

ADHD is one of the most common neurodevelopmental disorders, affecting 3–5% of school-age children. At least three times as many boys as girls are affected, and in clinically referred samples the ratio is often as high as 6:1. As many as one-third of people with ADHD may also meet the criteria for oppositional defiant disorder (ODD; see Chapter 5), and perhaps one-quarter of them eventually meet the criteria for conduct disorder (CD; Chapter 5).

Etiology

It has been known for a long time that ADHD runs in families. Strong evidence of genetic involvement has been derived from twin and adoption studies, in which about 50% of parents who themselves had ADHD have a child with the disorder, and 10–35% of children with ADHD have a first-degree relative with ADHD. It is common for parents, on being told that their child has ADHD, to realize that they themselves manifest the same syndrome. Although no individual predisposing genes for ADHD have been identified, molecular genetic studies have focused on chromosomal regions associated with dopamine pathways in the brain.

While there is ample evidence to support the existence of some abnormality of brain function, either genetic or acquired, environmental factors may also be involved. For example, ADHD is weakly linked to prematurity in the newborn. In any large sample of children with ADHD, prematurity is reported more often than would be expected, though most people with ADHD are not born prematurely.

Pathophysiology

Investigations of brain structure and function using advanced imaging devices have shown significant differences between healthy controls and patients with ADHD. Both noradrenergic and dopaminergic neuroreceptor systems have been implicated in the development of ADHD. The dopamine system acts in the brain in areas that are largely responsible for specific functions, such as the regulation of motor output. The noradrenergic system acts more broadly, controlling the state of arousal, selective attention and orientation, as well as the response to sensory stimulation.

Some evidence suggests that a subset of children with ADHD may also have sleep difficulties, but no definite link or causality in either direction has been established.

Long-term outcome

ADHD contributes to school failure and long-term difficulties in the workplace. The school problems are easy to understand: the child with ADHD usually has difficulty working alone or with groups, and finds it difficult to follow the teacher. Most symptoms of ADHD tend to improve with age, however, perhaps because people learn coping skills, and direct themselves into fields where their attention problems are less of an obstacle. Despite this, research indicates that 50–80% of children diagnosed with ADHD continue to experience symptoms into adulthood. In addition, much research suggests that adults with ADHD exhibit relatively high rates of depression and anxiety, and ADHD is associated with elevated alcohol and drug abuse.

Signs and symptoms

The three core symptoms of ADHD as defined in the *DSM-IV* are:

- hyperactivity
- impulsivity
- attention problems (Table 4.1).

These core symptoms manifest themselves in many different ways. For example, starting a task may be easy, but completing it may be very difficult for children with ADHD. They often break off what they are doing and impulsively move on to something else. These children may not be able to plan and see the whole, so they do not have a vision of a

TABLE 4.1

DSM-IV criteria for a diagnosis of ADHD

A. Either 1 or 2

1. Inattention

At least six of the following symptoms have persisted for at least 6 months to a degree that is maladaptive and inconsistent with developmental level

- Often fails to give close attention to details or makes careless mistakes in schoolwork or other activities
- Often has difficulty sustaining attention in tasks or play activities
- Often does not seem to listen to what is being said to him/her
- Often does not follow through on instructions and fails to finish schoolwork chores or duties in the workplace (not due to oppositional behavior or failure to understand instructions)
- Often has difficulty organizing tasks or activities
- Often avoids or strongly dislikes tasks such as schoolwork or homework that require sustained mental effort
- Often loses things necessary for tasks or activities, e.g. school assignments, pencils, books, tools or toys
- Often easily distracted by extraneous stimuli
- Often forgetful in daily activities

CONTINUED

TABLE 4.1 (CONTINUED)

2. Hyperactivity/impulsivity

At least six of the following symptoms have persisted for at least 6 months to a degree that is maladaptive and inconsistent with developmental level

Hyperactivity

- Often fidgets with hands or feet and squirms in seat
- Leaves seat in classroom or in other situations in which children are expected to remain seated
- Often runs about or climbs excessively in situations where it is inappropriate (in adolescents or adults this may be limited to feelings of restlessness)
- Often has difficulty playing or engaging in leisure activities quietly
- Is often on the go or often acts as if driven by a motor
- Often talks excessively

Impulsivity

- Often blurts out answers to questions before the questions have been completed
- Often has difficulty waiting in line or awaiting turn in games or group situations
- Often interrupts or intrudes on others

B. Onset no later than 7 years of age

C. Symptoms must be present in two or more situations, e.g. at school, at home, at work

D. The disturbance causes clinically significant distress or impairment in social, academic and/or occupational functioning

E. Does not occur exclusively during the course of a pervasive developmental disorder, schizophrenia, or other psychotic disorder, and is not better accounted for by a mood disorder, anxiety disorder, dissociative disorder or personality disorder

completed task, but rather see a task in fragmented parts, none of which relates to any others.

Assessment. ADHD cannot be identified by a single test. The diagnosis is a function of the frequency, severity and duration of the behaviors reported by the family. Two essential criteria for diagnosis are:
- the symptoms must have been present from a young age
- the child has to have the problems in more than one setting.

This is why it is important for both the parent and the doctor to make sure that there is a clear picture of how the child behaves at school, as well as at home.

It should be remembered that in different circumstances an individual's behavior can appear better or worse – trying to keep quiet in church is different from watching a football game. Children with ADHD are also known for the great variability in their patterns of behavior. They may show excessive attention in one situation, and then lack attention in other areas. This problem may reflect deficits in executive function rather than just attention. The child seems to lack inhibition and control.

Children can present with behavior that can be misdiagnosed as ADHD. Any of the conditions shown in Table 4.2 may coexist or present with similar symptoms. The differential diagnosis can be challenging in some cases, and is usually undertaken by a pediatrician or pediatric neurologist and a psychiatrist.

TABLE 4.2

Differential diagnosis of ADHD

- DCD
- Hearing problems
- Gilles de la Tourette's syndrome
- Trauma, including abuse
- Speech and language difficulties
- Dyslexia
- Asperger's syndrome

Evaluation of a child with suspected ADHD usually relies on rating scales for home and school in addition to the *DSM-IV* criteria. The Conners scale is best known and is one of the most consistent; it compares the child in school and at home to evaluate behavior patterns in different settings. Imaging and electroencephalography do not give sufficiently consistent results to be useful as diagnostic tools at present.

Treatment

Pharmacological treatment. At present the most common medical treatment, and the one that has been used for the longest time, is the central nervous system stimulant methylphenidate (Ritalin). It is started at a low dose and gradually increased to twice or three times daily. It is usually given after breakfast and after lunch, and its effect lasts for about 4 hours. Several long-acting, once-daily formulations are now on the market; these avoid the need for a midday dose at school and may have a better compliance profile. Dexamfetamine and imipramine can be used as well; risperidone and clonidine are also sometimes prescribed. All of these drugs must be prescribed under specialist supervision. Methylphenidate and dexamfetamine have been shown to be more effective than placebo. A recent meta-analysis of studies of short-acting methylphenidate, however, pointed out that all the studies were very short-term and many did not compare methylphenidate with placebo.

The side effects of stimulant medications can be troublesome (Table 4.3). The incidence of side effects is greater in children under 6 years of age, and this must be taken into account before starting treatment. Ongoing monitoring must be considered whenever drug treatment for ADHD is prescribed.

Psychosocial treatment. Various psychosocial and educational interventions can be helpful for children with ADHD, including:
- cognitive behavioral therapy
- behavior modification
- contingency treatment (e.g. reward systems, time-out) in school
- parent training in child management skills.

The last three types of treatment are more effective than cognitive

TABLE 4.3

Possible side effects of stimulant medications for ADHD

- Decreased appetite (the most prominent)
- Insomnia
- Stomach ache
- Drowsiness
- Dizziness

behavioral therapy in improving behavior and academic performance. There is little evidence to show that combined treatments are more effective than single therapy with medication, though combined treatments may have an effect on other symptoms, such as anxiety and social skills.

Underlying learning difficulties require additional individual or small group remedial instruction. Other allied health professionals may be involved in this; for example, an occupational therapist can offer specific programs for handwriting or gross motor difficulties, while a speech and language therapist can help with language difficulties.

Alternative treatment. Because pharmacologic or psychosocial treatments are not entirely satisfactory, many parents have sought alternative interventions for their children with ADHD. Unfortunately, many of the alternative treatments that have been promoted are not supported by empirical data. A review of such alternatives concluded that of the many therapies introduced and promoted for ADHD, nutritional intervention seemed to hold the most promise. Recent work in Canada suggests that amelioration of some of the mood symptoms often associated with ADHD is possible with broad-spectrum mineral and vitamin supplementation, but the use of such an intervention for the core symptoms of ADHD has yet to be tested.

Parent involvement in treatment. It is important not to underestimate the burden placed on families with a child (or several children) with

ADHD. Parenting and living with such children is far more challenging than living with a child with other school-based difficulties. This is probably particularly true for those families coping with a child whose ADHD is complicated by ODD, but this latter disorder has received very little attention from the research community. If parents are fully involved in their child's therapy, however, they can help to ameliorate difficult behaviors. Suggestions to help parents bringing up a child with ADHD are given in Table 4.4.

Cooperation between parents and teachers is essential for the management of any child with specific learning needs, but this seems to be particularly true for ADHD. Blaming staff or parents is counterproductive to addressing the child's needs within the resources that schools and home can provide.

School is often where children with ADHD face their greatest difficulties, and these children need to be supported at school with an

TABLE 4.4

Suggestions for parents of children with ADHD

- Develop consistent routines at home and school

- Keep rules clear and simple, and give reminders calmly

- Remember that your child does not intend to be difficult

- Try to redirect behavior

- Ensure you have your child's full attention when you are talking and keep reinforcing this; check that your child is making eye contact before giving instructions

- Supervise closely: impulsivity can place children in dangerous situations

- Be positive about your child; always look out for 'being good' and praise the child

- Try to ignore minor irritating behavior

- Provide clear disciplinary consequences: tell the child the rules, and if they are broken, be consistent about the consequence

- Allow your child 'time out', i.e. if the child feels out of control, remove him or her from the situation into a quiet, stimulus-free environment for a few minutes to cool off

educational program designed for their specific needs. A management plan should be developed in collaboration with teachers. Children with ADHD respond best to a highly organized and routine classroom structure, with a minimum of visual distraction and noise. They perform best if seated at the front of the room, as close to the class teacher as possible. Frequent adult input through the day may be necessary to keep the child on task, with opportunities for breaks to move around and burn off excess energy.

Key points – Attention deficit hyperactivity disorder

- ADHD is one of the most common neurodevelopmental disorders, affecting 3–5% of school-age children; at least three times as many boys as girls are affected.
- There is strong evidence that ADHD is genetically determined, but environmental factors may also be involved; it is also weakly linked to prematurity.
- Both noradrenergic and dopaminergic neuroreceptor systems have been implicated in the development of ADHD.
- Evaluation of a child with suspected ADHD usually relies on rating scales for home and school in addition to using the *DSM-IV* criteria.
- Treatment may be pharmacologic or psychosocial; alternative therapies have not yet been shown to be useful.
- CNS stimulants, in particular methylphenidate (Ritalin), are the most commonly prescribed drugs for treatment of ADHD.

Key references

Arnold LE. Treatment alternatives for attention-deficit/hyperactivity disorder (ADHD). *J Attention Disord* 1999;3:30–48.

Barkley RA. *Attention Deficit Hyperactivity Disorder: a Handbook for Diagnosis and Treatment.* 2nd edn. New York: Guilford Press, 1998.

Biederman J, Faraone SV, Spencer T et al. Patterns of psychiatric comorbidity, cognition, and psychosocial functioning in adults with attention deficit hyperactivity disorder. *Am J Psychiatry* 1993;150:1792–8.

Elia J, Ambrosini PJ, Rapoport JL. Treatment of attention-deficit-hyperactivity disorder. *N Engl J Med* 1999;340:780–8.

Fisher SE, Francks C, McCracken JT et al. A genomewide scan for loci involved in attention-deficit/hyperactivity disorder. *Am J Hum Genet* 2002;70:1183–96.

Kaplan BJ, Crawford SG, Gardner B, Farrelly G. Treatment of mood lability and explosive rage with minerals and vitamins: two case studies in children. *J Child Adolesc Psychopharmacol* 2002;12:205–19.

Kaplan BJ, Crawford SG, Dewey D, Fisher GC. The IQs of children with ADHD are normally distributed. *J Learning Disabil* 2000;33:425–32.

Kaplan BJ, Crawford SG, Fisher GC, Dewey DM. Family dysfunction is more strongly associated with ADHD than with general school problems. *J Attention Disord* 1998;2:209–16.

Kaplan BJ, Dewey D, Crawford SG, Fisher GC. Deficits in long-term memory are not characteristic of ADHD. *J Clin Exp Neuropsychol* 1998;20:518–28.

LaHoste GJ, Swanson JM, Wigal SB et al. Dopamine D4 receptor gene polymorphism is associated with attention deficit hyperactivity disorder. *Mol Psychiatry* 1996;1:121–4.

Rucklidge JJ, Kaplan BJ. Psychological functioning of women identified in adulthood with attention-deficit/hyperactivity disorder. *J Attention Disord* 1997;2:167–76.

Schachter HM, Pham B, King J et al. How efficacious and safe is short-acting methylphenidate for the treatment of attention-deficit disorder in children and adolescents? A meta-analysis. *CMAJ* 2001;165:1475–88.

5 Oppositional defiant disorder and conduct disorder

Most children at some point argue, talk back, disobey and defy parents and teachers. Oppositional behavior is often a normal part of a developmental stage for 2–3-year-olds and early adolescents. However, it is important to distinguish the pattern of oppositional defiant disorder (ODD) from the many children who are oppositional from time to time, particularly when they are tired, hungry, stressed or upset. Openly uncooperative and hostile behavior becomes a serious concern:

- when it is so frequent and consistent that it stands out in comparison with other children of the same age and developmental level
- when it affects the child's social, family, and academic life.

Conduct disorder (CD) is a more severe, repetitive and persistent pattern of behavior, in which the basic rights of others, or the major rules and values of society, are violated.

It has been estimated that 5–15% of all school-age children have ODD, with twice as many boys suffering from the condition than girls. In most studies the prevalence of CD is approximately 5% in the 10-year-old population, with a male-to-female ratio of 4:1.

Etiology

The causes of ODD are unknown, but many parents report that, from an early age, their child with ODD was more rigid and demanding than the child's siblings. Three variables have been statistically associated with negative outcomes in children with ODD:

- greater use of physical discipline by parents
- greater life stress for families
- more prenatal and perinatal complications.

The directionality of the influence of some of these variables must be questioned, of course. Few would suggest that the presence of ODD could cause perinatal complications, though underlying biological defects may possibly cause both birth-related complications and ODD.

The relationship between the other two variables (family stress and use of physical discipline) and ODD could be bidirectional.

Pathophysiology

It seems from the limited research so far carried out that there is not one single causative factor. In future, we hope diagnostic criteria will be restructured to capture adequate subtypes and indicators, the neurological underpinnings of the disorders will be clarified, and the models explaining the varied pathways to disruptive behavioral disorders will be refined on the basis of empirical research.

Gene studies looking at Gilles de la Tourette's syndrome, ADHD, stuttering, ODD and CD and other behaviors sometimes associated with Tourette's syndrome suggest that they are polygenic, due in part to three dopaminergic genes.

It seems likely that ODD/CD is influenced by additional genetic factors.

Long-term outcome

Some children with ODD progress to the more severe symptoms of CD, and others do not. Environmental, social and genetic influences appear to have an effect on outcome in individuals with ODD and CD. In boys, ODD is a strong risk factor for CD, while girls seem to have a greater increased risk of continued ODD, depression and anxiety.

The symptoms of CD are more often found in children of lower socioeconomic status from families with many problems; parental substance abuse, low socioeconomic status and oppositional behavior are key factors in the progression of ODD to CD. CD is apparently the only developmental behavioral disorder for which socioeconomic status is a significant predictor. In contrast to CD, the other difficulties reviewed in this book, such as dyslexia, ADHD and ODD itself, occur across all economic levels and appear to be independent of parental education and family function.

Substantial individual differences have been reported in the long-term outcomes for CD, ranging from worsening to sustained recovery, with most boys showing persistent but fluctuating levels of CD. In the research so far carried out, improvement in CD was not accounted for by treatment or incarceration. Predictors for a positive long-term outcome for CD are shown in Table 5.1.

Signs and symptoms

Children with ODD show an ongoing pattern of uncooperative, defiant and hostile behavior toward authority figures that seriously interferes with their day-to-day functioning. The *DSM-IV* criteria for the diagnosis of ODD are given in Table 5.2.

CD includes aggression to people and animals, property destruction, deceitfulness, theft, and severe violations of rules. The pattern may include stealing, intentional injury, and forced sexual activity. The diagnosis of CD according to the *DSM-IV* is made when the child exhibits a pattern of severe, repetitive, acting-out behavior, rather than an isolated, occasional incident (Table 5.3). Boys with CD are more inclined to fight, steal and participate in acts of vandalism, such as fire-setting. Girls with CD are more likely to lie, run away and be involved in severe sexual acting-out behavior, including prostitution. Both boys and girls with CD are at extremely high risk of substance abuse and problems at school.

ODD more commonly presents in school-age children, but may be tentatively diagnosed as early as 3 years of age. CD is almost never diagnosed in a child so young. ODD almost always precedes CD developmentally.

Assessment. A child presenting with oppositional symptoms should have a comprehensive assessment by a child and adolescent mental

---

TABLE 5.1

Predictors for a positive long-term outcome of CD

- Milder initial CD
- Fewer symptoms of attention deficit hyperactivity disorder
- Higher child verbal intelligence
- Greater family socioeconomic advantage
- Not having antisocial biological parents

TABLE 5.2

DSM-IV criteria for a diagnosis of ODD

A. A pattern of negativistic, hostile, and defiant behavior lasting at least 6 months, during which four (or more) of the following are present:

- Often loses temper
- Often argues with adults
- Often actively defies or refuses to comply with adults' requests or rules
- Often deliberately annoys people
- Often blames others for mistakes or misbehavior
- Is often touchy or easily annoyed by others
- Is often angry and resentful
- Is often spiteful or vindictive

Note: Consider a criterion met only if the behavior occurs more frequently than is typically observed in individuals of comparable age and developmental level

B. The disturbance in behavior causes clinically significant impairment in social, academic, or occupational functioning

C. The behaviors do not occur exclusively during the course of a psychotic or mood disorder

D. Criteria are not met for CD

Associated features

- Learning problem
- Depressed mood
- Hyperactivity
- Addiction
- Dramatic or erratic or antisocial personality

TABLE 5.3

DSM-IV criteria for a diagnosis of CD

For 12 months or more the patient has repeatedly violated rules, age-appropriate societal norms or the rights of others. This is shown by three or more of the following, at least one of which has occurred in the previous 6 months:

Aggression to people and animals

- Often bullies, threatens or intimidates others
- Often initiates physical fights
- Has used a weapon that can cause serious physical harm to others, e.g. a bat, brick, broken bottle, knife or gun
- Has been physically cruel to people
- Has been physically cruel to animals
- Has stolen while confronting a victim, e.g. mugging, purse snatching, extortion or armed robbery
- Has forced someone into sexual activity

Destruction of property

- Has deliberately engaged in fire-setting with the intention of causing serious damage
- Has deliberately destroyed others' property (other than by fire-setting)

Deceitfulness or theft

- Has broken into someone else's house, building or car
- Often lies to obtain goods or favors or to avoid obligations
- Has stolen items of non-trivial value without confronting a victim, e.g. shoplifting, but without breaking and entering, or forgery

Serious violations of rules

- Often stays out at night despite parental prohibitions, beginning before age 13 years
- Has run away from home overnight at least twice while living in parental or parental surrogate home (or once without returning for a lengthy period)
- Is often truant from school, beginning before age 13 years

health team. It is important to look for other disorders that may be present, including:

- ADHD
- learning disabilities
- mood disorders (depression, bipolar disorder)
- anxiety disorders.

There has been considerable debate over the ability to diagnose early symptoms of CD, bipolar disorder and ADHD, which may overlap. A multidisciplinary approach involving both education and health is essential if a coherent and consistent treatment plan is to be put in place. It may be difficult to improve the symptoms of ODD without treating any coexisting disorders.

Treatment

Some of the approaches to treatment of ODD are outlined in Table 5.4. A recent review has highlighted the need for primary care doctors to be aware of ODD and CD, in order to be able to provide brief, behaviorally focused parent counseling (Table 5.5) and pharmacotherapy, and to understand the referral routes for more intensive family and individual psychotherapy.

TABLE 5.4

Approaches to treatment of ODD

- Parent-training programs to help manage the child's behavior
- Individual psychotherapy to develop more effective anger management
- Family psychotherapy to improve communication
- Cognitive behavioral therapy to assist problem-solving and decrease negativity
- Social skills training to increase flexibility and improve frustration tolerance with peers

TABLE 5.5

Suggestions for parents of children with ODD/CD

- Always build on the positives, giving your child praise and positive reinforcement for flexibility or cooperation

- Take time out or a break if you are about to make the conflict with your child worse, not better. This provides a good model for your child. If your child decides to take time out to prevent overreacting, give support and praise

- Pick your battles. Because your child with ODD has trouble avoiding power struggles, prioritize the things you want your child to do. If you give your child time out for misbehavior, don't add time for arguing. Say 'Your time will start when you go to your room'

- Set up reasonable, age-appropriate limits with consequences that can be enforced consistently

- Maintain interests other than your child with ODD, so that managing your child doesn't take all your time and energy. Try to work with and obtain support from the other adults (teachers, coaches and spouse) dealing with your child

- Manage your own stress with exercise and relaxation. Use respite care as needed

- Give your child some choices so that the child's back isn't against the wall

- Recognize improvement, however small it may be

- Try to love your child despite the difficulties

Key points –
Oppositional defiant disorder and conduct disorder

- Children with ODD show an ongoing pattern of uncooperative, defiant and hostile behavior toward authority figures that seriously interferes with their day-to-day functioning.
- The behavior of children with CD includes aggression to people and animals, property destruction, deceitfulness, theft and severe violations of rules.
- It has been estimated that 5–15% of all school-age children have ODD, while the prevalence of CD is approximately 5% in the 10-year-old population; more boys than girls are affected by either condition.
- The causes of ODD are unknown, but poorer outcomes are associated with greater use of physical discipline by parents, greater life stress for families, and more prenatal and perinatal complications.
- In boys, ODD is a strong risk factor for CD, while girls seem to have a greater increased risk of continued ODD, depression and anxiety.
- CD is the only developmental behavioral disorder for which socioeconomic status is a significant predictor.
- A child presenting with oppositional symptoms should have a comprehensive assessment (including a search for other disorders) by a child and adolescent mental health team.
- Treatment approaches include parent-training programs, individual and family psychotherapy, cognitive behavioral therapy and social skills training.

Key references

Biederman J, Faraone SV, Milberger S et al. Is childhood oppositional defiant disorder a precursor to adolescent conduct disorder? Findings from a four-year follow-up study of children with ADHD. *J Am Acad Child Adolesc Psychiatry* 1996;35:1193–204.

Comings DE, Wu S, Chiu C et al. Polygenic inheritance of Tourette syndrome, stuttering, attention deficit hyperactivity, conduct, and oppositional defiant disorder: the additive and subtractive effect of the three dopaminergic genes – DRD2, D beta H, and DAT1. *Am J Med Genet* 1996;67:264–88.

Kim EY, Miklowitz DJ. Childhood mania, attention deficit hyperactivity disorder and conduct disorder: a critical review of diagnostic dilemmas. *Bipolar Disord* 2002;4: 215–25.

Lahey BB, Loeber R, Burke J, Rathouz PJ. Adolescent outcomes of childhood conduct disorder among clinic-referred boys: predictors of improvement. *J Abnorm Child Psychol* 2002;30:333–48.

Loeber R, Green SM, Keenan K, Lahey BB. Which boys will fare worse? Early predictors of the onset of conduct disorder in a six-year longitudinal study. *J Am Acad Child Adolesc Psychiatry* 1995;34: 499–509.

Nadder TS, Rutter M, Silberg JL et al. Genetic effects on the variation and covariation of attention deficit–hyperactivity disorder (ADHD) and oppositional–defiant disorder/conduct disorder (Odd/CD) symptomatologies across informant and occasion of measurement. *Psychol Med* 2002;32:39–53.

Rowe R, Maughan B, Pickles A et al. The relationship between DSM-IV oppositional defiant disorder and conduct disorder: findings from the Great Smoky Mountains Study. *J Child Psychol Psychiatry* 2002; 43:365–73.

Searight HR, Rottnek F, Abby SL. Conduct disorder: diagnosis and treatment in primary care. *Am Fam Physician* 2001;63:1579–88.

Speltz ML, Coy K, DeKlyen M et al. Early-onset oppositional defiant disorder: what factors predict its course? *Semin Clin Neuropsychiatry* 1998;3:302–19.

Asperger's syndrome was first described in four children by Hans Asperger in 1944. More recently in the UK, interest in the diagnosis was revived when it was used to describe a group of children similar to the original four. The American Psychiatric Association has classified Asperger's syndrome as a disorder in the *DSM-IV*, but here we will continue to refer to it as a syndrome. Many clinicians consider Asperger's syndrome to lie on the same continuum as autism, and include it in the umbrella description 'autistic spectrum disorders'.

Asperger's syndrome is a pervasive developmental disorder characterized by severe and sustained impairment in social interaction, in addition to restricted and repetitive patterns of behavior, interests and activities. These deficits affect socialization of the child in all situations and result in the individual lacking adaptability and flexibility, especially in new situations. In contrast to individuals who are more clearly autistic, people with Asperger's syndrome generally exhibit a relative preservation of language and cognitive abilities.

Asperger's syndrome occurs in approximately 4 per 1000 population, affecting at least four times as many boys as girls.

Etiology

Several theories have been proposed for the cause of Asperger's syndrome. One of these is based on the psychometric definition of males as individuals in whom systematizing is significantly better than empathizing (while females are defined as having the opposite cognitive profile). Using these definitions, Asperger's syndrome could be considered as an extreme of the normal male brain.

Although there is evidence for genetic factors playing a part in Asperger's syndrome, family studies have suggested that the expression and penetrance of the phenotype are variable. However, when examined along with autism and the autistic spectrum, Asperger's syndrome appears in the same families as do these other diagnoses, and may also be associated with families with schizoid personality disorder, non-verbal learning disabilities, and semantic–pragmatic disorder.

Pathophysiology

Some evidence has been obtained to support the existence of an abnormality in brain function in individuals with Asperger's syndrome. For example, positron emission tomography (PET) scanning shows that a highly circumscribed region of left medial prefrontal cortex does not seem to function in individuals with Asperger's syndrome in the same way as in the normal population. This area is known to be a crucial component of the brain system that underlies the normal understanding of other minds. Other studies implicate the cerebellum or the amygdala, while some report no differences from control subjects.

Long-term outcome

In the long term, individuals with Asperger's syndrome show higher levels of anxiety and obsessional symptoms than do individuals with CD. There is also an increased risk of depression, suicidal ideation, and explosive tempers compared with the normal population. These problems do require long-term surveillance to ensure that appropriate medical or psychological treatment is offered if required.

Individuals with Asperger's syndrome may lack the ability to integrate with peers, both in the workplace and socially, significantly handicapping their lives. This has been described as 'lifelong eccentricity'.

Signs and symptoms

The American Psychiatric Association criteria for diagnosis of Asperger's disorder are given in Table 6.1. Irrespective of whether the condition is considered to be a disorder or a syndrome, however, there is general agreement on the following characteristics:

- difficulty with social interaction
- difficulty with all aspects of communication
- obsessional traits
- narrow range of interests
- resistance to change, rigid

TABLE 6.1

DSM-IV criteria for a diagnosis of Asperger's disorder

A. Qualitative impairment in social interaction, as manifested by at least two of the following:
- Marked impairments in the use of multiple non-verbal behavior, such as eye-to-eye gaze, facial expression, body postures and gestures to regulate social interaction
- Failure to develop peer relationships appropriate to developmental level
- A lack of spontaneous seeking to share enjoyment, interests or achievements with other people, e.g. by a lack of showing, bringing or pointing out objects of interest
- Lack of social or emotional reciprocity

B. Restricted repetitive and stereotyped patterns of behavior, interests and activities, as manifested by at least one of the following:
- Encompassing preoccupation with one or more stereotyped and restricted patterns of interest that is abnormal in either intensity or focus
- Apparently inflexible adherence to specific, non-functional routines or rituals
- Stereotyped and repetitive motor mannerisms, e.g. hand or finger flapping or twisting, or complex whole-body movements
- Persistent preoccupation with parts of objects

C. The disturbance causes clinically significant impairments in other important areas of functioning

D. There is no clinically significant general delay in language, e.g. single words used by age 2 years, communicative phrases used by age 3 years

E. There is no clinically significant delay in cognitive development or in the development of age-appropriate self-help skills, adaptive behavior (other than social interaction) and curiosity about the environment in childhood

F. Criteria are not met for another specific pervasive developmental disorder or schizophrenia

- associated motor coordination difficulties
- no significant other language impairment
- pragmatic language dysfunction.

Pragmatics involve three major communication skills (Table 6.2). A child with pragmatic problems may have little variety in language use, may say inappropriate or unrelated things during conversations, or may tell stories in a disorganized way. The child may think too literally, may see things in a black-and-white manner, and may be seen by others as being 'too honest'. This may affect the child's ability to make and sustain friendships, especially in teen years, as a major means of communication for most teenagers is non-verbal.

Asperger's syndrome often overlaps with a number of other developmental disorders, including ADHD, ODD and OCD. The motor skills and coordination deficits inherent in DCD are also

TABLE 6.2

Impact of pragmatic language difficulties on communication

Communication skill	Difficulty experienced
Using language for different purposes, e.g. greeting, informing, demanding, promising and requesting appropriately	May find it harder to recognize sarcasm, idioms and metaphors
Being able to be adaptable and flexible with the use of language, e.g. being able to see how language should change according to the needs or expectations of a listener or situation	May use inappropriate language for the current situation, e.g. talking to friends is different from talking to headmaster or grandparent
Being able to cope in a changing situation, e.g. eating at home versus eating in a restaurant	Less adaptable and less flexible in ability to cope in differing settings; may not recognize facial gestures and subtle nuances of language in terms of tone and inference (also called *non-verbal learning difficulties*)

very often associated with Asperger's syndrome. The difficulties of assessing the overlap between these developmental disorders remains a challenge.

Diagnostic uncertainties. Currently there is some debate over the validity of the *DSM-IV* criteria for Asperger's disorder. Many researchers believe that there are insufficient data to differentiate Asperger's disorder from high-functioning autism, that is, the group of about 20% of individuals with autism who function in the normal or above-normal range of IQ.

There is also uncertainty about how the diagnosis of Asperger's syndrome relates to the North American concept of non-verbal learning disabilities, and these two may be very difficult to distinguish. On the other hand, combining the two terms may not be reasonable, because although Asperger's syndrome seldom exists without non-verbal learning disabilities, it is possible to have non-verbal learning difficulties without Asperger's syndrome.

Assessment. The length of time from suspicion to diagnosis may vary depending on local resources and the degree of impairment exhibited by the child, but it usually takes longer than a diagnosis of autism. The typical age at which autism may be screened is around 18 months, and the age at which a diagnosis can be made reliably is around 30 months of age. In contrast, Asperger's syndrome is not usually suspected, screened or confirmed until the child enters school. At present there is still limited community and professional knowledge in this area; this lack contributes to delays in both diagnosis and provision of appropriate support. An appropriate diagnosis of autism spectrum disorder may require a dual-level approach:

- routine developmental surveillance
- diagnosis and evaluation of autistic spectrum disorders to improve the rate of early suspicion and diagnosis, and therefore of early intervention.

Assessment is usually carried out by a multidisciplinary team based in a children's center or specialized autistic spectrum service. The individuals who may contribute to the team are listed in Table 6.3. Several

TABLE 6.3

Multidisciplinary team members for assessment of a child with suspected Asperger's syndrome

- Pediatrician
- Pediatric neurologist
- Child psychiatrist
- Psychologist
- Speech and language therapist
- Occupational therapist
- Educational psychologist

standardized tools may be used for assessment across the range of autistic spectrum disorders, including:
- the Diagnostic Interview for Social and Communication Disorders (DISCO)
- the Asperger Syndrome (and high-functioning autism) Diagnostic Interview (ASDI)
- the Childhood Asperger Syndrome Test (CAST).

Information from both school and home also contributes to the diagnosis.

Ideally, a child's understanding should be assessed in different environments to evaluate social interaction and to consider fully where there are deficits. The assessment also needs to determine the individual's specific profile, because of the high incidence of other, overlapping difficulties.

Treatment

There is sometimes confusion regarding which agency should provide care and whether it should come from 'health' or 'education' authorities. In fact, both are appropriate. In the shorter term, the child needs to be supported or given the skills to be able to access the school curriculum. Treatment in the longer term needs to address the social and communication difficulties that prevent the individual from leading an independent life.

Tailored treatment programs are required for each child with Asperger's syndrome, because of the heterogeneity of the social deficits that are found. A number of therapeutic models have been used for individuals with Asperger's syndrome, most of which require treatment in small groups or one-to-one. Many of the treatment programs for children are undertaken in a school setting with expert advice, or in specialist units. Parents can contribute by following the suggestions in Table 6.4.

Treatment approaches use a variety of tools, including

- Picture Exchange Communication System (PECS)
- Teaching and Education of Autistic Children and Handicapped Children (TEACH).

TABLE 6.4

Suggestions for parents of children with Asperger's syndrome

- Consider if there are any other overlapping developmental or learning problems
- Consider the environment, e.g. what supportive 'equipment' or approaches your child requires to be integrated into the class
- Consider how information is delivered to your child, ensuring that it is consistent in approach from one teacher to another and from home to school
- Help your child learn to reflect on his or her own behavior: give checking mechanisms for behavior and plan for future situations to increase the chances of success and to see if change may occur
- Role-play with your child to prepare for a new occasion
- Work on time concepts to help your child understand when something is going to change
- Use visual reminders to help prompt your child
- Use simple language, one instruction at a time; change may be slow
- Provide and create a supportive and sensitive environment
- Work on social distance and eye contact so your child is aware of how others may feel about his or her behavior

Key points – Asperger's syndrome

- Asperger's syndrome is a pervasive developmental disorder characterized by severe and sustained impairment in social interaction, in addition to restricted and repetitive patterns of behavior, interests and activities; it may lie on the same continuum as autism.
- Asperger's syndrome occurs in approximately 4 per 1000 population, affecting at least four times as many boys as girls.
- Asperger's syndrome may be an extreme of the normal male brain. There is also evidence for genetic factors playing a part in its etiology.
- An abnormality in the functioning of the left medial prefrontal cortex, which is involved with normal understanding of other minds, may underlie Asperger's syndrome.
- Although autism can be reliably diagnosed at around 30 months of age, Asperger's syndrome is not usually suspected, screened or confirmed until the child enters school.
- Assessment is usually carried out by a multidisciplinary team based in a children's center or specialized autistic spectrum service, using a range of standardized tools for autistic spectrum disorders.
- Ideally, a child's understanding should be assessed in different environments to evaluate social interaction and define the deficits; care must be taken to identify any other, overlapping difficulties.
- Tailored treatment programs are required for each child with Asperger's syndrome, because of the heterogeneity of the social deficits that are found.

PECS begins with teaching a student to exchange a picture of a desired item with a teacher, who immediately honors the request. Verbal prompts are not used, thus building immediate initiation and avoiding prompt dependency. The system goes on to teach discrimination of symbols, and then puts them all together in simple 'sentences'. Children are also taught to comment and answer direct questions. TEACH provides a systematic approach to learning and structure for the individual and is used with both children and adults.

Pharmacologic treatment. Although antidepressants, mood stabilizers, and other psychiatric medications are often used for symptomatic improvement of various associated behavioral and mood problems, Asperger's syndrome itself is not currently treatable pharmacologically. Most typically, a child may be given medication to deal with anxiety, depression, or ADHD symptomatology.

Key references

Attwood T. *Asperger's Syndrome: a Guide for Parents and Professionals.* London: Jessica Kingsley Publishers, 1998.

Baron-Cohen S. The extreme male brain theory of autism. *Trends Cogn Sci* 2002;6:248–54.

Burke JD, Loeber R, Birmaher B. Oppositional defiant disorder and conduct disorder: a review of the past 10 years, part II. *J Am Acad Child Adolesc Psychiatry* 2002;41: 1275–93.

Filipek PA, Accardo PJ, Baranek GT et al. The screening and diagnosis of autistic spectrum disorders. *J Autism Dev Disord* 1999;29:439–84.

Gillberg C, Gillberg C, Rastam M, Wentz E. The Asperger Syndrome (and high-functioning autism) Diagnostic Interview (ASDI): a preliminary study of a new structured clinical interview. *Autism* 2001;5: 57–66.

Gillberg C, Billstedt E. Autism and Asperger syndrome: coexistence with other clinical disorders. *Acta Psychiatr Scand* 2000;102:321–30.

Gillberg C, Nordin V, Ehlers S. Early detection of autism. Diagnostic instruments for clinicians. *Eur Child Adolesc Psychiatry* 1996;5:67–74.

Green D, Baird G, Barnett AL et al. The severity and nature of motor impairment in Asperger's syndrome: a comparison with specific developmental disorder of motor function. *J Child Psychol Psychiatry* 2002;43:655–68.

Green J, Gilchrist A, Burton D, Cox A. Social and psychiatric functioning in adolescents with Asperger syndrome compared with conduct disorder. *J Autism Dev Disord* 2000;30:279–93.

Happe F, Ehlers S, Fletcher P et al. 'Theory of mind' in the brain. Evidence from a PET scan study of Asperger syndrome. *Neuroreport* 1996;8:197–201.

Klin A, Volkmar, FR, Sparrow SS, eds. *Asperger Syndrome*. New York: Guilford Press, 2000.

Mayes SD, Calhoun SL, Crites DL. Does DSM-IV Asperger's disorder exist? *J Abnorm Child Psychol* 2001;29:263–71.

Scott FJ, Baron-Cohen S, Bolton P, Brayne C. The CAST (Childhood Asperger Syndrome Test): preliminary development of a UK screen for mainstream primary-school-age children. *Autism* 2002;6:9–31.

Tantam D. Asperger's Syndrome in adulthood. In: Frith U, ed. *Autism and Asperger Syndrome*. Cambridge: Cambridge University Press, 1991: 147–83.

Obsessive–compulsive disorder (OCD) is a potentially debilitating disorder in which the sufferer experiences recurrent and intrusive thoughts, ideas or impulses. The distress to young people caused by the characteristic intrusive, unwanted and often unpleasant thoughts or fears is commonly hidden, as children identify these symptoms as peculiar or embarrassing and keep them secret, sometimes for years. Similarly, compulsive behaviors, such as washing or checking, are usually perceived as unnecessary and often ridiculous, and children may go to great lengths to conceal them. As a result, many individuals diagnosed in adulthood with OCD report that their symptoms first began in childhood.

OCD in young people is common and under-recognized. Estimated prevalence rates in children and adolescents are about 1.5%. It occurs more in females than in males.

Etiology

OCD appears to run in families, but there is also an association with brain injury, Gilles de la Tourette's syndrome and motor tics. ADHD may coexist with OCD, and a prospective longitudinal study has shown long-term associations between tics, ADHD symptoms and OCD. Tics in childhood and early adolescence predict an increase in OCD symptoms in late adolescence and early adulthood. ADHD symptoms in adolescence predict more OCD symptoms in early adulthood, and OCD in adolescence predicts more ADHD symptoms in adulthood.

Pathophysiology

Imaging studies have revealed both structural and functional abnormalities in the basal ganglia. Significantly, OCD is one of the first psychiatric disorders in which both psychotherapy and drug treatment have been shown to reverse the functional metabolic changes.

Long-term outcome

In addition to causing acute distress and disruption to education and friendships, OCD in children can be highly disabling, associated with chronic psychiatric morbidity, as well as severe long-term social impairment. Evidence exists that early detection and treatment are important for minimizing the impairment experienced.

Signs and symptoms

Obsessions are persistent thoughts, impulses, or images that occur repeatedly and are experienced as intrusive, inappropriate, and distressing. The individual attempts to ignore or suppress the obsession or to neutralize it with some other thought or action, that is, a compulsion. Obsessions are not simply worries about real-life problems, and those affected recognize (at least at some point during the course of the disorder) that the obsessions are a product of their own minds. Some examples of typical obsessions are given in Table 7.1.

Compulsions are the repetitive behaviors that the individual feels driven to perform in response to an obsession or according to certain rigid rules. Compulsions are aimed at reducing discomfort or preventing some dreaded event, though they are clearly excessive or are unconnected in a realistic way to the event they are aimed to prevent (Table 7.2). For example, childhood compulsions may include avoiding

---

TABLE 7.1

Examples of obsessions

- Doubting obsessions, e.g. appliances, locks, written work
- Contamination obsessions, e.g. germs, bleach, AIDS, colors, death
- Aggressive obsessions, e.g. stabbing children, pushing loved ones into traffic
- Obsessions about accidentally harming others, e.g. contamination, poisoning, starting fires, running over pedestrians
- Sexual obsessions, e.g. disturbing sexual thoughts
- Other obsessions, e.g. blinking, songs or numbers stuck in head

TABLE 7.2

Examples of compulsions

- Washing and cleaning
- Checking
- Counting
- Repeating actions or thoughts
- Hoarding
- Symmetry and exactness
- Repeating words, phrases, or prayers to oneself

stepping on cracks in paving stones and a belief that some awful event will occur if the child does step on a gap. Children may switch a light on and off a certain number of times, or until it 'feels right', or repeat a phrase (or ask the parent to repeat it) until it 'sounds right'. Symmetry, order, routine, touching and counting may also be features.

If asked directly, children can often give clear accounts of their problems, which are easily distinguished from ordinary childhood superstitions or rigidity of behavior. A diagnosis of OCD is made if the symptoms fulfill the criteria of the American Psychiatric Association *DSM-IV* (Table 7.3). Symptoms may come and go, however, and improve or worsen over time.

TABLE 7.3

DSM-IV **criteria for a diagnosis of OCD**

The OCD symptoms:

- Cause clinically significant distress or functional impairment (e.g. take more than 1 hour per day)
- Are not better accounted for by another disorder
- Are not better accounted for by a general medical condition or use of a substance

Assessment. A proper diagnosis usually requires a referral to a child psychiatrist, and a child and adolescent mental health team. Assessment is usually qualitative in nature and is based on the symptoms and signs reported by the child and family. A thorough clinical history is the most important aspect of a proper diagnosis. Structured interviews, such as the Yale–Brown Obsessive–Compulsive Scale, can be employed clinically to assess the severity of the symptoms.

Treatment

At least 70–80% of children with OCD are likely to respond to treatment with medication and behavioral therapy. To target treatment appropriately, children with OCD need careful evaluation to rule out normal developmental variations, depression, and autistic disorders, and to thoroughly assess their symptom severity and consequent impairment. Therapy also needs to be linked to school to ensure sufficient support is given to the child.

Behavioral therapy. A behavioral approach involves a detailed assessment of the problem, often starting with the child and family keeping a diary of the obsessions and compulsions. The aim of the treatment is to teach young people how to gain control of the problem by tackling it a little bit at a time. Behavioral therapy usually needs to take place over several sessions, and improvement may take several months. Treating additional symptoms, such as anxiety, depression and tic disorders, is also important to improve the success rate.

Informed parents can help too (Table 7.4); they may wish to read some of the books listed in Table 7.5.

Medication. Current medications used for the treatment of OCD include clomipramine, fluvoxamine, paroxetine and fluoxetine. These medications can help to diminish obsessive thinking and the subsequent compulsive behaviors. However, the US Food and Drug Administration has noted that there may be a link between some antidepressant drugs, including fluvoxamine, paroxetine and fluoxetine, and suicidal ideation or suicide attempts in pediatric patients. Such drugs should be used at the lowest dose consistent with good patient management.

TABLE 7.4

Suggestions for parents of children with OCD

- Recognize that your child cannot help many of the behaviors and rituals
- Try to recognize the behaviors and rituals, as your child may otherwise 'hide' them from you
- Try to improve your child's self-esteem
- Ensure your child takes prescribed medication regularly
- Support your child and plan carefully for transition points that may worsen the anxiety and OCD symptoms, e.g. change of school, going on holiday
- Create routine in the day so that your child feels safe and knows what will be happening

TABLE 7.5

Useful reading for parents

- Judith Rapoport. *The Boy Who Couldn't Stop Washing*. New York: Penguin Books, 1989
- Katharine A Phillips. *The Broken Mirror*. New York: Oxford University Press, 1996
- J Jay Fruehling. *Drug Treatment of OCD in Children and Adolescents*. North Branford, CT: Obsessive–Compulsive Foundation, 1997
- Tamar Chansky. *Freeing Your Child from Obsessive–Compulsive Disorder*. New York: Crown, 2000
- Fred Penzel. *Obsessive–Compulsive Disorders: A Complete Guide to Getting Well and Staying Well*. New York: Oxford University Press, 2000
- Constance H Foster. *Polly's Magic Games* (a book for children). Ellsworth, Maine: Dilligaf Publishing, 1994

Nutritional supplementation. Although no alternative treatment approach to OCD has been adequately studied or supported, an interesting case report suggests the possibility of ameliorating obsessional thoughts with broad-based nutrient supplementation.

Key points – Obsessive–compulsive disorder

- OCD is a disorder in which the sufferer experiences recurrent and intrusive thoughts, ideas or impulses (obsessions), which are often neutralized by compulsive behaviors.
- OCD in young people is common and under-recognized, with estimated prevalence rates in children and adolescents of about 1.5%; it occurs more in females than in males.
- OCD appears to run in families, but there is also an association with brain injury, Gilles de la Tourette's syndrome and motor tics; ADHD commonly coexists.
- Imaging studies have revealed both structural and functional abnormalities in the basal ganglia, and both psychotherapy and drug treatment can reverse the functional metabolic changes.
- Diagnosis usually requires a referral to a child psychiatrist, and a child and adolescent mental health team; assessment is usually qualitative, though a clinical rating scale may be used to assess the severity of symptoms.
- At least 70–80% of children with OCD are likely to respond to treatment with medication and behavioral therapy.
- Current medications used for the treatment of OCD include clomipramine, fluvoxamine, paroxetine and fluoxetine, all of which can help to diminish obsessive thinking and consequent compulsive behaviors.

Key references

Bolton D, Luckie M, Steinberg D. Long-term course of obsessive–compulsive disorder treated in adolescence. *J Am Acad Child Adolesc Psychiatry* 1995;34: 1441–50.

Geller DA, Biederman J, Faraone SV et al. Attention-deficit/hyperactivity disorder in children and adolescents with obsessive–compulsive disorder: fact or artifact? *J Am Acad Child Adolesc Psychiatry* 2002;41:52–8.

Kaplan BJ, Crawford SG, Gardner B, Farrelly G. Treatment of mood lability and explosive rage with minerals and vitamins: two case studies in children. *J Child Adolesc Psychopharmacol* 2002;12:205–19.

Leonard HL, Swedo SE, Lenane MC et al. A 2- to 7-year follow-up study of 54 obsessive–compulsive children and adolescents. *Arch Gen Psychiatry* 1993;50:429–39.

McGuire PK. The brain in obsessive–compulsive disorder. *J Neurol Neurosurg Psychiatry* 1995;59:457–9.

March JS, Mulle K, Herbel B. Behavioral psychotherapy for children and adolescents with obsessive–compulsive disorder: an open trial of a new protocol-driven treatment package. *J Am Acad Child Adolesc Psychiatry* 1994;33:333–41.

Peterson BS, Pine DS, Cohen P, Brook JS. Prospective, longitudinal study of tic, obsessive–compulsive, and attention-deficit/hyperactivity disorders in an epidemiological sample. *J Am Acad Child Adolesc Psychiatry* 2001;40:685–95.

Rasmussen SA, Eisen JL. Epidemiology of obsessive compulsive disorder. *J Clin Psychiatry* 1990;51(suppl):10–13.

Scahill L, Riddle MA, McSwiggin-Hardin M et al. Children's Yale–Brown and Obsessive Compulsive Scale: reliability and validity. *J Am Acad Child Adolesc Psychiatry* 1997;36:844–52.

Swedo SE, Leonard HL, Garvey MA et al. Pediatric autoimmune neuropsychiatric disorders associated with streptococcal infections (PANDAS): a clinical description of the first fifty cases. *Mol Psychiatry* 2002;7(suppl 2):S24–5.

Valleni-Basile LA, Garrison CZ, Jackson KL et al. Frequency of obsessive–compulsive disorder in a community sample of young adolescents. *J Am Acad Child Adolesc Psychiatry* 1994;33:782–91.

A world consensus is growing that more children with developmental problems are presenting themselves to physicians than was once the case. This increase has considerable implications in three major areas:

• increased demand on primary care time
• greater symptom complexity
• increased service needs.

These are some of the challenges that must be overcome for the next decade if the needs of children with developmental disorders are to be met.

Increased demands on primary care time

As more children appear in family physicians' offices, these physicians must become experts in areas not represented in their medical training. They must learn to recognize the signs and symptoms and to understand educational assessments, occupational therapy treatments and many more aspects of specific learning difficulties.

Greater symptom complexity

When the American Psychiatric Association published the third edition of the *Diagnostic and Statistical Manual* 20 years ago, there was no doubt that ADHD existed as a disorder, but there was considerable debate surrounding the issue of subtyping. The subtyping was brought clearly into focus in the fourth edition of the *DSM*, published in 1994. Even a cursory glance at the published literature now, however, reveals that the primary issue is no longer the nature of ADHD itself, but rather the increasing complexity of ADHD, the so-called 'comorbidities'. In other words, ADHD is now seen as part of a complex constellation of psychiatric problems that includes the mood and anxiety disorders.

The challenge for the physician is to understand that developmental disorders are no longer seen as little islands of impairment. Rather, each individual is truly unique, with an idiosyncratic bundle of symptoms.

Some symptoms will fit neatly into a psychiatric category, but it is likely that the individual patient will not. We often use diagnostic labels to provide an easier way of describing sets of symptoms to our patients, but they may also artificially compartmentalize the individual and oversimplify the developmental disorders, and thus the treatment approaches. Good diagnostic tools are an essential component in understanding functional difficulties.

Increased service needs

As both parents and professionals become more aware of the developmental disorders, and as symptom presentation becomes increasingly complex, there will be an inevitable increase in the needs for various services. For example, if children's needs are to be met and families appropriately supported, information gained from research must be applied in everyday practice in both the health and educational arenas.

The worldwide shortages in trained professionals in all areas can lead to frustration for parents. If demands for services are to be sufficiently met, then models of practice must be sought that lead to efficient and effective interdisciplinary working, in order to combine precious skills. This must be the gold standard that we should all aim to meet. Multidisciplinary work requires an openness in considering models of practice across disciplines in both primary and secondary care and in education. Children with developmental disorders require an approach based on communication between all parties, including the child and the parents.

Useful addresses

General information

Learning Disabilities Association
of America
4156 Library Road
Pittsburgh, PA 15234-1349, USA
Tel: 412 341 1515
Fax: 412 344 0224
www.ldanatl.org

Learning Disabilities Association
of Canada
323 Chapel St.
Ottawa, Ontario K1N 7Z2,
Canada
Tel: 613 238 5721
Fax: 613 235 5391
E-mail: information@ldac-taac.ca
www.ldac-taac.ca

SNAP (Special Needs Advisory
Project) Cymru
10 Coopers Yard
Curran Road
Cardiff, CF10 5NB, UK
Tel: 029 20 388776
Fax: 029 20 371876
E-mail: info@snapcymru.org
www.snapcymru.org

Network 81
1–7 Woodfield Terrace
Stansted
Essex, CM24 8AJ, UK
Tel: 0870 770 3262
Helpline: 0870 770 3306
(Mon–Fri 10.00–14.00)
Fax: 0870 770 3263
E-mail: network81@tesco.net

SANE (UK)
Tel: 020 7375 1002
SANEline: 0845 767 8000
(Mon–Sun 12.00–14.00)
www.sane.org.uk/

MIND (UK)
Tel: 08457 660163
Fax: 020 8522 1725
E-mail: contact@mind.org.uk
www.mind.org.uk

DCD

Dyscovery Centre
4A Church Road
Cardiff, CF14 2DZ, UK
Tel: 02920 628222
www.dyscovery.co.uk

The Dyspraxia Foundation
West Alley
Hitchin
Herts, SG5 1EG, UK
Tel: 01462 454986
www.dyspraxiafoundation.org.uk

Dyslexia

The British Dyslexia Association
98 London Road
Reading, RG1 5AU, UK
Tel: 0118 966 2677
Helpline: 0118 966 8271
Fax: 0118 935 1927
E-mail: admin@bda-
dyslexia.demon.co.uk
info@dyslexiahelp-
bda.demon.co.uk
www.bda-dyslexia.org.uk

**The International Dyslexia
Association**
Chester Building, Suite 382
8600 LaSalle Road
Baltimore, Maryland 21286-
2044, USA
Tel: 410 296 0232 (Mon–Fri
8:30–16:30 EST)
Fax: 410 321 5069
Requests for information: 1 800
ABCD123
www.interdys.org/index.jsp

ADHD

**CHADD (Children and Adults
with ADHD) USA**
8181 Professional Place, Suite 201
Landover, MD 20785, USA
Tel: (800) 233 4050 or 301 306
7070
Fax: 301 306 7090
www.chadd.org

CHADD Canada
1376 Bank Street
Ottawa, Ontario, K1H 7Y3
Canada
Tel: 613 731 1209
Fax: 604 272 6651
E-mail: info@chaddcanada.org
www.chaddcanada.org

The National Attention Deficit Disorder Association
1788 Second Street, Suite 200
Highland Park, IL 60035, USA
Tel: 847 432 ADDA
Fax: 847 432 5874
E-mail: mail@add.org
www.add.org

ADD/ADHD Family Support Group
Mrs Gillian Mead (President)
1a The High Street
Dilton Marsh
Nr Westbury
Wiltshire, BA13 4DL, UK

Hyperactive Children's Support Group
Ms Sally Bunday
71 Whyke Lane
Chichester
West Sussex, PO19 2LD, UK
Tel: 01903 725 182
Fax: 01903 734 726
www.hacsg.org.uk

ODD and CD
Tough Love International (TLI)
Post Office Box 1069
Doylestown, PA 18901, USA
Tel: 800 333 1069
Fax: 215 348-9874
E-mail: service@toughlove.org
www.toughlove.org
www.conductdisorders.com
www.behaviour.org.uk

Asperger's syndrome
Asperger Syndrome Coalition of the US
PO Box 351268
Jacksonville, FL 32235-1268, USA
Tel: 1 866 4 ASPRGR
www.asperger.org/support/support _main.html

OASIS (Online Asperger Syndrome Information and Support)
www.udel.edu/bkirby/asperger/

Autism

The National Autistic Society
393 City Road
London EC1V 1NG
UK
Tel: 020 7833 2299
Fax: 020 7833 9666
E-mail: nas@nas.org.uk

Afasic
2nd Floor
50–52 Great Sutton Street
London, EC1V 0DJ, UK
Tel: 020 7490 9410
Fax: 020 7251 2834
Email: info@afasic.org.uk
www.afasic.org.uk

I-CAN
4 Dyer's Buildings
Holborn
London, EC1N 2QP, UK
Tel: 0870 010 4066
Fax: 0870 010 4067

OCD

Anxiety Disorders Association of America
8730 Georgia Ave, Suite 600
Silver Spring, MD 20910, USA
Tel: 240 485 1001
Fax: 240 485 1035
www.adaa.org

Obsessive–Compulsive
Foundation, Inc.
337 Notch Hill Road
North Branford, CT 06471, USA
Tel: 203 315 2190
Fax: 203 315 2196
E-mail: info@ocfoundation.org
www.ocfoundation.org

OCD Action (UK)
Tel: 020 7226 4000
www.ocdaction.org.uk

Index

aggression and vandalism 44,
45, 48
alcohol and drug abuse 32,
42, 43, 44
American Psychiatric
Association 4, 5, 24, 50,
51, 67
anger management 46
Asperger Syndrome
Diagnostic Interview (ASDI)
4, 55
Asperger's syndrome 5, 7–8,
9, 35, 50–9
assessment 54–5
diagnostic difficulty 54
DSM-IV criteria 52, 54
etiology 50–1
genetic factors 50–1, 57
long-term outcome 51
pathophysiology 51
pragmatic language
difficulties 53
prevalence 50, 57
signs and symptoms 51–4
suggestions for parents 56
treatment 55
typical problems 50, 51, 52,
53, 57
assessment and diagnosis 5,
9–10, 13
see also specific difficulties
by name
Aston Index 19
attention deficit disorder
(ADD) 4, 5, 31–40
see also ADHD
attention deficit hyperactivity
disorder (ADHD) 4, 5, 8, 9,
27, 31–40, 42, 43, 46, 53,
58, 60, 65, 67
assessment 35–6
differential diagnoses 34, 35
DSM-IV criteria 33–4,
36, 39
etiology 31–2
genetic factors 31–2, 39
long-term outcome 32

management plan 38–9
pathophysiology 32
prevalence 31, 39
signs and symptoms 33–6
suggestions for parents 37–9
treatment 36–9
typical problems 33–5
atypical brain development
8, 9
autistic spectrum disorders
50, 54, 57, 63

ball skills 9, 26
baseline assessment 7
behavior modification 36–7,
63, 65
brain injury 60
British Dyslexia Association
15

causes 5
see also specific difficulties
by name
cerebral palsy 9, 27
child management skills
training 36–7
Childhood Asperger
Syndrome Test (CAST) 4, 55
clinical observations 9
clinical psychologists 11
clomipramine 63, 65
clonidine 36
CNS stimulants 36, 37, 39
cognitive behavioral therapy
28, 29, 36–7, 46
comorbidity 8, 67
concentration problems 9
conduct disorder (CD) 4, 5,
31, 41–9
assessment 46
diagnosis 46
DSM-IV criteria 45
genetic factors 42
long-term outcomes 42–3
pathophysiology 42
prevalence 41
signs and symptoms 43

suggestions for parents 47
treatment 46–7
connective tissue disorder
25, 29
Conners scale 36
contingency treatment 36–7
coordination skills 24, 25, 26,
29, 53

depression and anxiety 32,
34, 37, 42, 46, 48, 51,
58, 63
antidepressants 58
developmental coordination
disorder (DCD) 4, 5, 8, 9,
24–30,
35, 53–4
assessment 27–8, 29
differential diagnoses 25, 27
DSM-IV criteria 27
etiology and
pathophysiology 24–5, 29
long-term outcome 25
prevalence 24
signs and symptoms 25–8
suggestions for parents
28, 29
treatment 28–9
typical problems 25–7
dexamfetamine 36
Diagnostic and Statistical
Manual of Mental
Disorders, 4th edition
(DSM-IV) 4, 5, 9, 31
Diagnostic Interviews for
Social and Communication
Disorders (DISCO) 4, 55
diagnostic labels 13, 68
advantages 7
disadvantages 7–8
versus functional labels 8–9
differential diagnosis 9
see also specific difficulties
by name
dissociative disorder 34
dopamine pathways 32, 39
DSM-IV criteria 4

see also specific difficulties by name
dyslexia 4, 5, 7, 8, 9, 15–23, 27, 35, 42
  assessment 17–20, 21
  DSM-IV criteria 17, 18
  etiology 15–16
  genetic factors 15, 16, 21
  intervention 15, 20
  long-term outcome 16
  pathophysiology 16
  prevalence 15, 21
  remediation programs 18–19, 20, 21
  signs and symptoms 16–20
  suggestions for parents 20–1
  treatment 20–1
  typical problems 17, 19, 21
Dyslexia Early Years Screening Test 4, 19
Dyslexia Screening Test (DST) 4, 19
dyspraxia see developmental coordination disorder

educational psychologists 18, 19, 20, 21, 29, 55
Ehlers–Danlos syndrome 25
electroencephalography 36
environmental factors 32, 39, 42
epilepsy 9
etiology see causes

family dysfunction 11
fluoxetine 63, 65
fluvoxamine 63, 65
formal testing 9
functional labels 9, 13
funding 7
future trends 67–8

genetic factors 15, 16, 21
  see also specific difficulties by name
Gilles de la Tourette's syndrome 35, 42, 60, 65

handwriting 9, 37
  see also DCD; dyslexia
hemiplegia 27

high-functioning autism 54
hyperactivity–impulsivity 31, 33–5, 38
hypotonic problems 25, 29

imaging 36, 60, 65
imipramine 36
improvement 11
impulsive behavior 9
  see also hyperactivity
inattention 31, 33, 35, 39
incidence 5
  see also specific difficulties by name
inhibition 35
intervention focus 7, 13
  see also specific difficulties by name

labeling children 7–9
Learning Disabilities Association 13
legal reference point 7
lifelong eccentricity 51
local educational services
  in North America 12–13
  in the UK 12

management 10–12
  at home 5, 13
  in school 5, 12–13
  individualized plan 11, 13
  see also specific difficulties by name
methylphenidate (Ritalin) 36, 39
mineral and vitamin supplementation 37
mood disorder 34, 67
mood stabilizers 58
motor coordination disorder 27, 28
motor skills 24, 25, 29, 53
  fine 24, 26
  gross 24, 28, 29, 37
motor tics 60, 63, 65
multidisciplinary approach 9–10, 13, 54, 55, 57, 63, 65, 68
multisensory treatment 20, 21

muscular dystrophy 9, 27
myopathic disorder 25, 29
myotonic disorder 25, 29

neurofibromatosis 25
neurological disorders 9, 10, 39
neuromuscular problems 25, 29
non-verbal learning disabilities 51, 53, 54
noradrenergic system 32, 39
nutritional intervention 37, 64

obsessive–compulsive disorder (OCD) 4, 5, 53, 60–6
  assessment 63
  DSM-IV criteria 62
  etiology 60
  genetic factors 60, 65
  long-term outcome 61
  pathophysiology 60
  prevalence 60, 65
  signs and symptoms 61–3, 65
  suggestions for parents 63, 64
    useful reading 64
  treatment 63–4, 65
  typical behavior patterns 61, 62, 65
occupational therapists 11, 24, 28, 29, 37, 55
oppositional defiant disorder (ODD) 4, 5, 8, 31, 38, 41–9, 53
  assessment 43, 46
  DSM-IV criteria 43, 44
  etiology 41–2
  genetic factors 42
  long-term outcome 42–3
  pathophysiology 42
  prevalence 41, 48
  signs and symptoms 43
  suggestions for parents 47
  treatment 46–7
  typical behavior patterns 43, 44, 45
overlapping conditions 8, 13, 27, 43–4, 56, 57

parent support organizations
13
parents
advantages of diagnostic
labels 7
practical advice 12, 46, 48
see also specific difficulties
by name
parents' observations 10, 55,
63
paroxetine 63, 65
pediatric neurologists 11, 35,
55
pediatricians 11, 35, 55
peer relationships 11
personality disorder 34
pharmacologic treatment 36,
39, 46, 58, 60, 65
side-effects 36, 37, 39
physiotherapists 11, 29
Picture Exchange
Communication System
(PECS) 4, 56, 57-8
positron emission tomography
(PET) 51
prematurity 32, 39
prevalence 5
see also specific difficulties
by name
primary care team 11, 13,
67
processing difficulties 15, 16,
18, 19-20, 21
progress review 11
psychiatrists 35, 55, 63,
65
psychosocial treatment 36-7,
39
psychotherapy 46, 60, 65
psychotic disorder 34

reading disability see dyslexia
recurrent intrusive
thoughts/impulses 60, 61, 65
remediation programs
at home 10
in school 7, 10
see also specific difficulties
by name
research inclusion 7
risperidone 36

schizoid personality disorder
51
schizophrenia 34, 52
self-esteem 11, 25, 64
hobbies to encourage 29
semantic–pragmatic disorder
51
service delivery 7
service needs increase 67, 68
social relationship problems 9,
11, 50, 51, 52, 57
social skills training 46, 48
socioeconomic status and CD
42, 48
special educational needs
coordinator (SENCO) 4, 12,
20
specialist services 7, 11–12, 13
speech and language therapists
11, 18, 20, 37, 55
spelling problems see dyslexia
sports suitable for
coordination disorder 29
stuttering 42
suicidal ideation 51
symptoms and signs 5
greater complexity 67–8
see also specific difficulties
by name

teachers' observations 10
Teaching and Education of
Autistic Children and
Handicapped Children
(TEACH) 4, 57, 59
trauma 35, 60, 65
treatment 5
individualized programs 8,
10, 56, 57
see also specific difficulties
by name

voluntary organizations 12, 13

waiting lists 11–12
Wechsler Individual
Achievement Test II (WIAT
II) 4, 19
Wechsler Intelligence Scale for
Children, version III (WISC
III) 4, 18–19

Woodcock–Johnson
Psychoeducational Battery –
revised (WJ–R) 4, 19

Yale–Brown
Obsessive–Compulsive Scale
63